The Future of Age-Based
Public Policy

9,101

The Future
of Age-Based
Public Policy

Edited by
ROBERT B. HUDSON

THE JOHNS HOPKINS UNIVERSITY PRESS
Baltimore and London

© 1997 The Johns Hopkins University Press
All rights reserved. Published 1997
Printed in the United States of America on acid-free paper
06 05 04 03 02 01 00 99 98 97   5 4 3 2 1

The Johns Hopkins University Press
2715 North Charles Street
Baltimore, Maryland 21218-4319
The Johns Hopkins Press Ltd., London

Earlier versions of chapters 2 through 9 and 11 through 16 appeared in *Generations* 19,
no. 3 (1995), the journal of the American Society on Aging. Chapter 3 is adapted, with
permission, from an article of the same title that first appeared in *Policy Paper No. 10*
(December 30, 1994), a publication of the National Taxpayers Union. Chapter 10 is
excerpted from testimony presented before the Senate Finance Committee Subcommittee
on Social Security and Family Policy on March 25, 1996; the views are those of the
author and do not necessarily reflect the views of Watson Wyatt Worldwide or any of
its other associates.

Library of Congress Cataloging-in-Publication Data will be found at the end of
this book.
A catalog record for this book is available from the British Library.

ISBN 0-8018-5659-0
ISBN 0-8018-5660-4 (pbk.)

Contents

Contributors

Paul Adams, D.S.W., Professor, Graduate School of Social Work, Portland State University, Portland, Oregon

Robert Applebaum, Ph.D., Professor, Department of Sociology, and Research Fellow, Scripps Gerontology Center, Miami University, Oxford, Ohio

Robert H. Binstock, Ph.D., Professor of Aging, Health, and Society, Department of Epidemiology and Biostatistics, School of Medicine, Case Western Reserve University, Cleveland, Ohio

Francis G. Caro, Ph.D., Director of Research, Gerontology Institute, University of Massachusetts, Boston, Massachusetts

Gary L. Dominick, Doctoral Candidate, Graduate School of Social Work, Portland State University, Portland, Oregon

Judith G. Gonyea, Ph.D., Associate Professor and Chair, Department of Social Research, School of Social Work, Boston University, Boston, Massachusetts

Martha Holstein, Ph.D., Research Scholar, Park Ridge Center for the Study of Health, Faith, and Ethics, Chicago, Illinois

Neil Howe, M.A., M.Ph., Chief Economist, National Taxpayers Union Foundation, Washington, D.C.

Robert B. Hudson, Ph.D., Professor and Chair, Department of Social Welfare Policy, School of Social Work, Boston University, Boston, Massachusetts

Diane E. Justice, M.A., Deputy Director, National Association of State Units on Aging, Washington, D.C.

Eric R. Kingson, Ph.D., Associate Professor, Graduate School of Social Work, Boston College, Chestnut Hill, Massachusetts

Elizabeth A. Kutza, Ph.D., Director, Institute on Aging, School of Urban and Public Affairs, Portland State University, Portland, Oregon

Robert Logan, M.A., Executive Director, Council on Aging of the Cincinnati Area, Cincinnati, Ohio

Marilyn Moon, Ph.D., Senior Fellow, Urban Institute, Washington, D.C.

Robert Morris, D.S.W., Cardinal Medeiros Visiting Lecturer, Gerontology Institute, University of Massachusetts, Boston, Massachusetts

John Myles, Ph.D., Professor, Department of Sociology, Florida State University, Tallahassee, Florida

Jill Quadagno, Ph.D., Professor of Sociology, Pepper Institute of Aging and Public Policy, Florida State University, Tallahassee, Florida

Anna M. Rappaport, F.S.A., Managing Director, William M. Mercer, Incorporated, Chicago, Illinois

Sylvester J. Schieber, Ph.D., Vice President, Watson Wyatt Worldwide, Washington, D.C.

Monika White, Ph.D., President and Executive Director, Senior Health and Peer Counseling, Santa Monica, California

Preface

This book addresses one of the most pressing issues facing U.S. social policy as we approach the turn of the century: What should be our public posture toward an older population that is growing in numbers and in diversity? The past quarter-century has seen remarkable progress in improving the life circumstances of older Americans, but this progress has been accompanied by public expenditures that are both very significant and growing rapidly. Indeed, the questions surrounding age-based policy today center more on curtailing eligibility for programs and benefits than on expanding them. The purpose of this volume is to examine the political, population, policy, and programmatic issues and options associated with the future of age-based policy.

The Future of Age-Based Public Policy is the reworking, expansion, and updating of an issue of *Generations,* the journal of the American Society on Aging, devoted to the same topic and for which I served as guest editor. That issue, including contributions from most of the authors found here, appeared in the summer of 1995. Later that year, Robert H. Binstock, consulting editor in gerontology to the Johns Hopkins University Press, approached me about expanding and updating the *Generations* issue in book form. After further consultations with Wendy Harris, medical editor at the Press, and reviews by referees, there was agreement to move forward with the project. Authors were pleased with the opportunity to rework their contributions—especially in the light of events since their manuscripts had been prepared—and new submissions were readily forthcoming. In addition to very much appreciating the support of all these parties in making this book a reality, I would like to thank Mary Johnson, staff editor of *Generations,* for her extensive efforts in giving this project its initial form and focus.

In the opening chapter, I provide a context for addressing age-based public policy. The chapter reviews the historical and political rationales for so heavily featuring advanced age in our social policies. It then itemizes a series of policy reforms that would render policies for aged people more selective or more inclusive. The chapter concludes by presenting population and program data, detailing the ways in which public policy has recognized the needs and the contributions of older people.

The book is then organized into four parts. The first, "The Competing Bases for Policy Benefits," contains four chapters articulating competing rationales for policy allocations. Martha Holstein, a social ethicist, presents a compelling case for the use of age as a criterion for eligibility. Taking a far different approach, Neil Howe calls attention to what he sees as the unsustainable growth in age-based and age-related policies and cites the need for drastically curtailing such expenditures. While also not subscribing to age as a determining factor, John Myles goes in the opposite direction from Howe, making the case for universality and "social citizenship," that is, the case for extending benefit beyond old people, not cutting benefits to old people. The part's concluding chapter, by Robert Binstock, reviews the politics of age-based policy and the posture of age-based interest groups, especially the American Association of Retired Persons, toward these issues.

The book's second part, "Public Policy and Population Dynamics," explores the policy dilemmas being generated by emergent demographic trends in today's and tomorrow's America. Judith Gonyea assesses the situation of the fastest-growing population in the United States, the oldest old, seeing high levels of need but, as well, much more diversity than is conventionally associated with that population. Robert Morris and Francis Caro tackle issues associated with yet another emergent older population, the young old, paying particular attention to the ability of this group, through both work and voluntarism, to contribute to society as well as to receive from it. Finally, Paul Adams and Gary Dominick address relations between young people and old people, emphasizing the in-kind contributions represented by rearing the children who will later support old people and whose well-being must be ensured so that they are able to perform that role.

Part III, "Policy Arenas and the Place of Age," systematically reviews the issues associated with the major public policies in place benefiting older people. Eric Kingson and Jill Quadagno characterize many of the efforts to transform Social Security as being less about Social Security itself than about generating a "crisis mentality" directed at public sector intervention more generally. Sylvester Schieber has a very different perspective on the Social Security question, and his contribution here is an outline of how we might partially privatize the program and, over time, transform it into one that is fully funded rather than funded on a so-called pay-as-you-go basis. Marilyn Moon reviews the arguments for and against maintaining Medicare as confined largely to old people, observing that the overall health profile of elderly people may justify the continuation of Medicare as an age-based program distinct from other private or public insurance programs that might be created. Elizabeth Kutza turns our attention to the place of old people in the Medicaid program, centering her concerns on issues of fairness within this means-tested program and using program innovations in Oregon to concretize her observations. Community long-term care for old people has made great strides in recent years, and Diane Justice reviews that progress and the issues of targeting benefits and sharing costs so that limited resources might be made widely available. With so much attention being paid to the rise of private sector initiatives in aging, Anna Rappaport depicts the shifting roles of employer and employee in the provision of private pension and health care benefits, emphasizing efforts by employers to limit their obligations to employees and to place greater responsibility on employees for making choices and assuming risks.

The book concludes with part IV, "Two Case Studies," that reviews the experiences of community long-term care programs in two states. Robert Logan and Robert Applebaum examine Hamilton County (Cincinnati), Ohio, and the program undertaken in the wake of a county levy passed to support services for people over sixty years of age. In partial contrast, Monika White discusses the experiences under California's Linkages program, which was designed to serve functionally impaired adults of all ages. The authors review the political rationales behind age-based and non-age-based programs and the initial implementation experiences with each program. By contrasting these two initiatives, the book comes back to its central theme, the pros and cons of using advanced age as a major, if not singular, rationale for the receipt of public policy benefits.

The Future of Age-Based
Public Policy

1

The History and Place of Age-Based Public Policy

ROBERT B. HUDSON

Provisions benefiting older people have long been a hallmark of social policy in the United States. Given their life circumstances, it is perhaps not surprising that aged persons receive a far greater volume of public benefits than do younger populations. Social policy in the United States is nonetheless distinctive because it allocates a higher proportion of social welfare expenditures to old people than do other industrial nations, it employs age as an eligibility criterion more than is the case elsewhere, and in using chronological age, the United State puts greater emphasis on the needs of the old than on those of the young.

Old Age a Policy Variable

There are compelling reasons, both historical and current, to recognize advanced age as a major variable in social policy. The most obvious is that age has long stood as a formidable proxy for demonstrable need and, in turn, for the receipt of social support from the larger society. Indeed, old age was long understood—in addition to illness, disability, and unemployment—to be one of the "bad things" (Rubinow 1934) that can happen to people in industrial society.

In the United States, greater recognition has been given to old age as a bad thing than to other risks or contingencies associated with modern life. Outliving one's income was long the most dire prospect facing old persons. That prospect was far from remote, given that, as recently as sixty years ago, at least half of older people are estimated to have been poor and that some three-quarters of income in old age came from one's adult children (Brody 1987). Few would have argued with Franklin Roosevelt's contention, made while governor of New York, that "poverty in old age should not be regarded either as a disgrace or necessarily as a result of lack of thrift or energy. Usually it is a mere by-product of modern industrial life" (Rimlinger 1971, 212). However, thanks largely to Social Security's Old Age and Survivors Insurance (OASI) program, income insecurity among old people has declined dramatically. Poverty rates have dropped, median incomes have increased, and the proportion of income that elders receive from family members has plummeted to a current estimate of only 2 percent. Supporters and critics alike acknowledge the enormous contribution OASI has made.

With the passage of time, improvements on the income front, and the growth of the older population, access to health care was the next issue to move to center stage. Older people played two critical roles in the federal government's launching of a national health insurance program. First, older people had great need for expanded health care coverage—only roughly one-half of the elderly population had any form of private health care coverage at the time of Medicare's enactment in 1965. Second, older people were critical politically. In a country in which individuals were largely expected to take care of themselves, they were, in Marmor's (1970, 17) well-known words, "one of the few population groupings about whom one could not say the members should take care of their financial-medical problems by earning and saving more money." In America's "reluctant welfare state" (Wilensky and Lebeaux 1965, xii), sympathies toward the old, rather than clashes among social classes, were required to usher in broad-based, publicly funded, health care insurance.

Finally, advanced age as a basis for policy benefits has extended itself to the world of public assistance. That Old Age Assistance was Title I of the 1935 Social Security Act is less surprising than what happened in the early 1970s, when Old Age Assistance and analogous programs for blind and disabled persons were reorganized into the Supplemental Security Income (SSI) program. In nationalizing these programs and providing the nation's first guaranteed income, SSI was unquestionably a positive step in the annals of public welfare. Yet the policy process that ultimately yielded SSI in 1973 began as an attempt by the Nixon administration to significantly restructure the Aid to Families with Dependent Children program by replacing it with the Family Assistance Plan. Then as now, however, such controversy surrounded any expansion of benefits for young adult welfare recipients and their children—especially one involving income guarantees—that the only aspect to be salvaged from the entire effort was the creation of such a guarantee for the adult categories (i.e., SSI for poor old, blind, and disabled persons; see Burke and Burke 1974).

In addition to old age having long been a proxy for need, it has also been a meaningful marker of an inability to work. That presumption, in turn, necessitated the enactment of provisions for retirement income. Over the course of the mid-twentieth century, the basis for making that provision evolved "from relief to income maintenance" (Heclo 1974). This important conceptual shift was in the direction of seeking to replace a percentage of prior earnings rather than providing a more modest minimum amount to simply ward off destitution. Until as recently as the early 1950s, there existed a struggle between these two approaches, one favoring the expansion of the means-tested public assistance programs, and the other favoring the expansion of the earnings replacement approach found in OASI and based on workers' wages and contributions. That, today, expenditures under OASI approach ten times those under the old-age portion of SSI shows the social insurance approach to have clearly carried the day. In so doing, it also established the commitment to maintain some percentage of workers' incomes when they could no longer work.

The presumed (or enforced) inability of old persons to work also contributed to the later enactment of health insurance for old people (Medicare) because private health insurance in the United States is provided overwhelmingly through employment. Over time, OASI greatly improved the ability of elders to meet what might be considered ordinary consumption needs (e.g., food, housing, transportation), but it certainly did not provide enough to cover the costs of major illnesses, and the private insurance market did not choose to extend to retirees the health insurance coverage that made available to workers. Thus, Medicare was enacted to fill this void and to help protect the modicum of economic security retirees had begun to enjoy.

How appropriate old age remains as a proxy for negative events is central to any discussion of the future of age-based benefits. Clearly, growing numbers of very affluent elders do not "need" Social Security, and growing numbers of educated and healthy elders have the capacity

to work. Both of these are very significant developments and lie behind current proposals to partially means-test and privatize benefits
for old persons or to "remake" age a better proxy by raising the age of
eligibility for benefits.

Indeed, even the benefits discussed to this point are not based on
age alone. Most benefits for old people are based, as well, on need or
demonstrated (and recorded) contributions rendered by an individual
over decades of paid work and social activity. The Social Security benefit formula concretizes the linkage between work and benefits. The
amount received is related directly to the amount contributed, reflecting the underlying value of equity. But there is also an adjustment in
the formula, giving a higher return on contributed dollars to lower-
income workers, reflecting the value of adequacy. As well, the indexing of initial Old Age Insurance benefits to the wages of current
workers is a means of formally acknowledging the efforts made by
today's retirees earlier in life.

These earlier contributions of older people can also be recognized
more broadly and symbolically than through documented contributions. Nelson (1982) refers to the recognition that can be accorded an
older individual on the grounds of "veteranship." Former Social Security Commissioner Robert Ball (1985), one clearly knowledgeable
about the ways of the Federal Insurance Contribution Act (FICA),
pays homage to the societal contributions made throughout a working
life: "We owe much of what we are to the past. We all stand on the
shoulders of generations that came before. They built the schools and
established the ideals of an educated society. They wrote the books,
developed the scientific ways of thinking, passed on the ethical and
spiritual values, discovered our country, developed it, won its freedom,
held it together, cleared its forests, built its railroads and factories and
invented new technologies." Richard Leone of the Twentieth Century
Fund concurs in Ball's assessment, noting that "even the debt a new
generation must pay off is accompanied by the government bonds and
other assets that it inherits" (Leone 1996, 15).

Age-Related Policy Today: Success or Excess?

Recent and quite extraordinary events have placed age-based policy in
a far different context from what was the case in 1935, or 1965, or
even 1975. In sum, these events have taken heretofore noncontroversial policy allocations devoted to old persons and subjected them to

hard scrutiny and, from some quarters, intense criticism. These events are serving to recast the politics of aging; the degree to which they will (and should) transform age-based policies remains to be determined.

Newfound Well-Being among Old People

Perhaps the most striking of these transformations is the heightened aggregate well-being among old people that has been achieved since the 1960s. No longer can it be said that old people are universally needy or, as was historically nearly the case, singularly needy. Poverty among old persons has declined by a factor of three since the late 1950s, from nearly 40 percent to the current 12.2 percent. Alarmingly, poverty among children has been rising since the 1970s, to a point where, at 22.7 percent, it is nearly double that of older people (U.S. Bureau of the Census 1992). The broader aging population has made notable economic progress in recent decades, as well. Among households headed by people age sixty-five or older, inflation-adjusted income increased from $8,940 in 1967 to $15,143 in 1992, or 69 percent; in comparison, the rise in median income among younger households was 26 percent over the same time span (Radner 1996). The role of Social Security in these developments is seen in a study by the U.S. Bureau of the Census (1988), which concludes that social insurance programs, principally Social Security, has done more to alleviate poverty and inequality among old people than either the tax system or other social programs, including welfare.

There is also a new twist on the matter of older Americans' ability to work. While it was long common knowledge that older people "couldn't work," in fact, they did. As recently as 1950, labor force participation rate among older men was 46 percent, a figure that has until very recently fallen steadily, to the point at which only about 16 percent of older men were working in 1991. The pattern for women, however, is largely unchanged over recent decades, "the combined effects of increased participation by women and decreased participation by the elderly" (Quinn and Burkhauser 1990). Nonetheless, beginning at age sixty-two, when early Social Security benefits may be taken, participation in the labor force falls off sharply. Due in part to improved health but especially to the availability of retirement income through Social Security, fewer older people today *must* work than has historically been the case.

Improved well-being among old people is now generating renewed interest in having older people work or contribute to society either through paid employment or in some other manner. One manifestation of encouraging increased participation in the labor force among old people is the 1995 liberalization of the so-called earnings test under Social Security. Under this legislation, the amount that older persons (between age sixty-five and sixty-nine) can earn without any offset to their Social Security benefits will increase from $11,280 in 1995 over the next several years until it is capped at $30,000. Proponents of the change argue that older people should not be discouraged from working by imposing a high added "tax" on their Social Security benefits. Critics argue that raising the exempt amount to include all moderate and some higher income undermines the principal intent of OASI, namely, to aid those no longer working. Herein, of course, lies the crux of the issue: Is it that people cannot work and, therefore, must be supported through an income maintenance program, or is that people can work and should not be discouraged from doing so through offsetting benefits against earnings?

Another manifestation of the newfound abilities among today's old people is captured under the rubric of "productive aging." Old people should no longer be viewed as people in need of support after their "useful" life has ended but, rather, as a population whose wisdom and energy can make great contributions to society. As suggested by the liberalization of the earnings test, many believe that continued work by the elderly population should be encouraged. As noted by Schulz (1995), however, there are at least two formidable barriers to increased full-time employment among older adults: many of them do not wish to work in regular, full-time jobs, and many employers do not wish to hire them. One way of acknowledging both of these concerns is addressed by those who encourage both older people and employers to design part-time, flexible work schedules, perhaps at lower pay scales than those offered middle-aged workers. Such secondary labor market participation is not without its critics—why should older workers be compensated differently from younger workers?—but such opportunities are growing in the private economy. Whether they take the form of secondary labor activity or simple voluntarism, there are jobs to be done—literacy projects, work with low-income children, environmental efforts—and growing numbers of healthy, active, and educated elders able to perform them.

Cast more broadly, these observations highlight the recent appearance of an older population never before seen: "the young old" (Neugarten 1974), "the able old" (Morris and Bass 1988), and a "third age" (Laslett 1987). Through the use of a "third-age indicator" (a 0.5 or greater probability that persons, having attained age twenty, will live to age seventy, and that at least 10% of the population is age sixty-five or older), Laslett documents that the third age, which was nowhere a "majoritarian reality" before the twentieth century, became a settled feature of the industrial nations in the 1980s. Put differently, the third age represents the first time in history that there are large numbers of older people whose existence is centrally defined neither by work nor by illness. The presence of such a population raises fundamental questions about the shape and purpose of a host of social policies and certainly puts the criterion of age in a heretofore unseen light.

This remarkable progress notwithstanding, there remain pressing economic and social problems among old people. That many of these problems are associated with a fourth age—in which very old women, with low incomes, in frail health, and nearly socially invisible, are found disproportionately—makes them in some ways more stark rather than less. The needs of the population in the fourth age are perhaps best seen in data related to chronic illness, functional impairment, and the use of institutional and community services. People over age eighty-five are five times more likely to be disabled or impaired than those age sixty-five through seventy-four (LaPlante and Miller 1992). Women over age sixty-four account for 80 percent of older people living alone (Kasper 1988), and women represent 75 percent of nursing home residents (Dolinsky and Rosenwaike 1988). When race is added to age and gender as correlates of need, income differentials among old people are the sharpest. Older women are twice as likely to be poor as older men, older black men are five times more likely to be poor than older white men, and 9.7 percent of persons age sixty-five through seventy-four are currently poor, in contrast to 16 percent of persons age seventy-five and older. Combining age, race, and gender creates the most stunning contrast, virtually a tenfold disparity: the poverty rate among white men age sixty-five through seventy-four is 4.5 percent; the poverty rate among black women age seventy-five and older is 43.9 percent (U.S. General Accounting Office 1992).

No longer does the gerontological community need to convince people that there are wide differentials in well-being among old people. Given that, historically, elders almost inevitably lived in dire straits makes this new diversity (i.e., the impressive growth in numbers of older persons who live in relatively comfortable circumstances) a welcome development. Yet, in a time of governmental retrenchment, this diversity does pose major questions for public policy and especially for age-based public policies.

Intergenerational Issues

A spate of material has appeared in recent years presenting evidence that the success of current policies in addressing the needs of elders will increasingly come at the expense of younger and future generations. Lamm and Lamm (1996) acknowledge that the contributions of Social Security and Medicare "deserve our respect" but argue that if these programs continue to go untouched "with taxes as high as 60 percent of each paycheck, the next generation will have little incentive to work." Kotlikoff (1996) also sees a dire future for the young and the unborn. For generations born throughout the twentieth century, lifetime net tax burdens have risen moderately, from 24 percent for those born in 1900 to 34 percent for those born in 1993. He estimates, however, that the comparable rate for future generations may run as high as 84 percent. To right this generational imbalance, we would have to either cut income taxes by 41 percent beginning in 1996 or cut Social Security, Medicare, and other federal transfer payments by 30 percent.

While others find these estimates either extreme or, as is often said of futures research, inherently unreliable, all parties to the debate over age-related spending realize that changes must be made in Social Security and Medicare if they are to remain secure. Thus, former Social Security Commissioner Ball suggests that Social Security could remain sound well into the next century but only if we (1) extend coverage to state and local workers not in the system, (2) reduce benefits by 3 percent by computing them over thirty-eight years instead of thirty-five years, (3) tax all benefits that exceed what the worker has paid in, and (4) increase the return on the Social Security trust funds by investing a portion of them in corporate securities (Jones 1996). These certainly are modest reforms compared to those derived from Kotlikoff's calculations. But if one remembers that only twenty years ago, any taxation of Social Security benefits was considered political suicide (Stockman 1975), it is clear how rapidly concern about Social Security (and Medicare) is moving from broadening coverage and expanding benefits to preserving programs while not violating norms of equity, whether by income or by generation.

Clearly, the fates of people who are old at different points in time will vary depending on the generations they belong to. It may, in fact, turn out that the current generation of older people will be judged to have won in this "generational roulette." In a cross-national examination of several industrial countries, Thomson (1989) argues that today's old people may represent a "welfare generation." These individuals were young earlier in the century at a time when the welfare state itself was young. In those early years, many of the benefits centered on education and housing, areas in which children and young adults were disproportionate beneficiaries. Over time, as the welfare state aged, these individuals aged as well. By the 1970s, and certainly since, welfare state benefits were increasingly directed toward old people, primarily in the areas of pensions and health care. Thomson does not argue that this shift was by design or due to some pernicious selfish political influences, but he does suggest that this generation—born roughly between the two world wars—may turn out to have benefited considerably more from governmental programs than the generations that preceded it and that will follow it.

At least insofar as age-based policies are concerned, generation has now joined class, gender, and age itself as a quality-of-life indicator. The life-course perspective, once largely the province of social psychology, has now entered policy debates, if not necessarily by that name. Important cross-sectional comparisons (the well-being of older people and children at any point in time) will now be joined by longitudinal ones (the costs and benefits to different generations—when they are both young and old—over the course of time).

Whither (Wither?) the Public Sector?

A third trend forcing a reconsideration of age-based policy is less about policy than about government itself. A rising tide of conservative commentary, analysis, and advocacy, beginning in the mid-1970s, has succeeded in placing debate about the role, size, and purpose of the federal government very much at the center of the political stage. For President Clinton to have spoken of "ending welfare as we know it" and to have said that "the era of big government is over" is an indicator of how discourse about policy and government has shifted to the right.

Age-based programs, because of their size, have been very much caught up in this trend, but these programs are more fodder than targets. True, attempts by the ascendent congressional Republican majority throughout 1995 to reduce Medicare spending by $270 billion and

Medicaid by $180 billion over seven years were billed as efforts to "save" the programs in the long run and to reduce the federal budget deficit, but reining in the federal government itself was on the agenda, as well. Quadagno (1996) argues that conservative commentators have transformed both rising program expenditures and growing governmental deficits into an "entitlement crisis." In the absence of dramatic reductions in spending, enormous public sector expenditures for these programs will stifle needed economic growth and leave today's children facing onerous and unjust burdens. The "crisis" is as much about the responsibilities of and expectations for the federal government as it is about expenditures and deficits.

The emergence of this ideological debate, centered on the role of government, places age-based and age-related programs in a new light. In the period circa 1965–74, "you couldn't do enough for older people." In the 1980s, tax cuts, defense outlays, and rising entitlement expenditures combined to generate very sizable budget deficits and to constrain program growth. Today, policies directed toward old people are caught up in a battle of public sector legitimacy. It is in this context, rather than in one centered on either demography or deficits, that proposals to means-test or privatize Social Security and Medicare must be understood. The outcome is far from certain, but the terms of the debate are fundamentally different from what they were ten or twenty years ago.

Alternatives and Adjuncts to Age as a Policy Criterion

In the United States, advanced age has unquestionably been an important threshold for the receipt of policy benefits. Yet, with rare exception, attaining a given age has been necessary but not sufficient for the receipt of those benefits. For example, both Old Age Insurance and Medicare impose age thresholds but also require an employment history with covered earnings; age-based benefits under Supplemental Security Income and Medicaid necessitate that one also be poor; Employee Retirement Income Security Act protections presuppose that one's employer offered pension benefits in the first place; publicly supported elder housing programs invariably involve a formal means test. The only clear exceptions to this necessary-but-not-sufficient condition are found in the Older Americans Act and in legislation regarding age discrimination, in which age and interpretations of it are central.

Exclusion Efforts

The presence of multiple eligibility conditions for old people introduces important subtleties into the debate about the future of so-called age-based programs. If age should assume a lesser place in the overall determination of eligibility, what should substitute for it? Heightened economic and functional means testing, the partial privatization of programs, and raising the age of eligibility for benefits have each been actively advanced in recent years.

The means testing of income and assets is definitionally at the heart of public assistance programs, most notably SSI and Medicaid in the case of aged people. The success of Social Security in improving the economic situation of older people has contained expenditure growth in the age-based provisions of SSI, but SSI is a critical supplement for low-income elders with minimal or low-paying work histories. Medicaid has evolved into a program of enormous importance for low-income frail elders, funding virtually one-half of all nursing home expenditures in the United States. Many Medicaid beneficiaries receive SSI (all SSI recipients are eligible for Medicaid), but others "spend down" to meet "medically indigent" eligibility standards. In the absence of a social insurance program for chronically ill and functionally impaired elders (and others), Medicaid has become the locus of such care.

Another form of mean testing found under so-called Medicaid waiver and "state-only" programs for community long-term care services is cost sharing. Usually through a sliding-scale fee mechanism, participants are asked or required to cover some portion of the cost of services. Initial fears that such fees would discourage low-income and minority populations to participate have been shown to be largely ill founded, and these programs (which do not currently include the Older Americans Act, where cost sharing continues to be prohibited) have continued to expand. Indeed, participants report that being able to contribute to these costs makes them feel more self-reliant. It may be that cost sharing resonates differently from other forms of means testing in that it has both the consequence and the aura of expanding rather than shrinking the eligibility pool.

So-called functional means testing has also received increased attention in recent years as a way to heighten the target efficiency of health and social service programs for older people. The dramatic increases in expenditures for long-term care in both institutional and community settings have led to widespread introduction of functional impairment criteria, most notably scales that assess the performance of activities of daily living, or ADLs. Where used appropriately, broad-scaled client assessments can result both in cost savings—limiting services to persons with several ADL "deficits"—and in promoting equity—ensuring that individuals with comparable impairments receive the same level of service. Case management procedures at the clinical level and managed care structures within the larger financing and delivery system both center on functional means testing (Hudson 1996).

More remarkable than income and functional means testing and cost sharing for public assistance and service programs are proposals to means-test Social Security. A hallmark of Social Security to this point has been that benefits are based solely on work history, independent of any other income or wealth considerations. Even subjecting a portion of high-income beneficiaries' benefits to income taxation does not violate this spirit; it simply states that this income through Social Security should be considered comparable to other income sources for tax purposes. In contrast, the Concord Coalition—headed by former Senators Paul Tsongas and Warren Rudman and investment banker Peter Peterson—proposed an "affluence test" for Social Security (and selected other entitlement programs). In their proposal, reductions in benefits would be phased in when household income exceeded $40,000. The proportion of benefits withheld would increase with income, the top tier being households with incomes in excess of $120,000, which would lose 85 percent of the benefits to which they are entitled under current law.

If need is the only test, imposing an affluence test on rich people makes eminent sense. Imposing, at least at the top levels, a nearly confiscatory tax on benefits would not violate needs-based criteria. The difficulty with the plan lies more on the equity side of the equation, namely, high-income individuals facing high marginal tax rates on their benefits will have little reason to stay in the system. With political support eroding among higher-income (and influential) individuals, the system might well splinter, creating a "means-avoiding" system. The loss of higher-income participants would also erode the ability of the system to provide a higher rate of return to lower-income retirees than is possible through their contributions alone.

A yet more radical approach to restructuring Social Security centers on proposals to partially privatize the system. Based on the belief that individuals should have more control over the major assets associated with retirement and that the current pay-as-you-go system contains serious intergenerational inequities, these plans would, over time, transform much of Social Security into publicly mandated but privately owned accounts. In proposals put forth by Gramlich (forthcoming) and by Schieber (1996), all workers would contribute to a pooled, first-tier, minimum-benefit account, not unlike Social Security today. Above that amount, however, contributions would be deposited into one's own personal retirement account. By placing recipients in different systems—even with some overlap—the Gramlich and Schieber proposals would fundamentally restructure the universal OASI program. Inferentially, the plans say that no longer are the income risks faced by all older people sufficiently similar to warrant their remaining in a common program. The positive aspect of this in historical terms is that such proposals would concretize the belief that many older people are sufficiently able, educated, and well off to no longer require a paternalistic federal program. The plan would, however, notably segment recipient populations. Lower-income people would be entirely or largely in the first benefit tier, and while higher-income persons would also be found there, their economic and psychic presence would be relatively meaningless in the light of the accumulations in their private accounts.

A final option under consideration in some circles, raising the age for the receipt of age-based benefits (notably Social Security and Medicare), expressly reendorses advanced age as a criterion of eligibility for benefits, now by simply pushing up the age thresholds. Indeed, by concentrating attention on the "older old" within the aged population, it brings back to the fore the need and inability-to-work criteria as core rationales for eligibility. Current law calls for raising the age for full Social Security benefits to sixty-six early in the next century and to sixty-seven by 2027, and a proposal by Senators Kerrey and Simpson would accelerate that schedule. Policy issues associated with raising the age of eligibility for benefits include concern about how moderately disabled older workers (not eligible for disability benefits) would fare (Moon and Mulvey 1996) and whether, in fact, employers would hire those now presumed by policy to be employable.

There are, as well, broader-based value concerns that should be brought to the discussion of raising the age for benefit eligibility. On the one hand, limiting benefits to the older old would heighten target efficiency centered on need and would do so with the administrative simplicity that a chronological age brings with it. But very advanced age is a less precise proxy than is often assumed (see Gonyea, this volume). More philosophically, this increased targeting of benefits might come at a high price to individual and population dignity. Put differently, do we, in some way, negate the progress made over seven decades in improving the lot of old people by redefining old age to be, once again, a residual life stage marked by poverty, illness, and dependency (Hudson 1988)?

Inclusion Efforts

Alternatives to the age-based policies prominently featured in the United States are also found in proposals that are more, rather than less, inclusive. Indeed, the development of the modern welfare state in most industrial nations was based on some combination of class-based politics and at least limited endorsement of the idea of social citizenship. Such beliefs hold that certain substantive benefits should be afforded to society's members by virtue of their citizenship rather than by virtue of either need (public assistance) or work effort (social insurance). Despite pressures on social welfare programs throughout the industrialized world, most contemporary welfare states continue "to alter or offset the outcome of market transactions" and "provide income or services that are not dependent on the outcome of market exchanges" (Brown 1988, 4).

The United States and Australia are frequent exceptions to even elastic cross-national generalizations about the development of the welfare state. One well-known indicator developed by Esping-Andersen (1990) centers on decommodification, that is, how well individuals eligible for social welfare benefits fare economically when circumstances take them out of the labor market. Using an index based on eligibility, income replacement rates, and range of entitlements, Esping-Andersen rank-ordered industrial nations, as shown in table 1.1.

The position of the United States in such a ranking should come as no surprise; it has long been considered an exception in its "reluctance" to develop an institutionalized social welfare structure (Wilensky and Lebeaux 1965). Esping-Andersen's threefold categorization finds the United States as part of a "liberal" welfare state history, in contrast to "corporatist" ones found in central Europe and "universalist" ones, which Scandinavian systems come closest to approximating. Indeed, that the very idea of insurance, to say nothing of social

Table 1.1.
The Rank Order of Welfare States, by the Decommodification Index, 1980

Country	Score [a]
Australia	13.0
United States	13.8
New Zealand	17.1
Canada	22.0
Ireland	23.3
United Kingdom	23.4
Italy	24.1
Japan	27.1
France	27.5
Germany	27.7
Finland	29.2
Switzerland	29.8
Austria	31.1
Belgium	32.4
Netherlands	32.4
Denmark	38.1
Norway	38.3
Sweden	39.1
Mean	27.2
Standard deviation	7.7

Source: Esping-Andersen (1990).
[a] Index is based on eligibility, income replacement rates, and entitlements.

insurance, was suspect in the United States until the latter portion of the nineteenth century (Lowi 1990) is but one indicator of how removed much U.S. thinking has been from both collective and public interventions.

At a point in time when European regimes are moving in the direction of heightened "commodification," there is little reason to expect that the United States will move toward more inclusive approaches to eligibility and benefits. In fact, as suggested earlier, advanced age served as something of an ideological loss leader in helping expand the U.S. welfare state to where it is today. That role has now passed, having given way to the multiple concerns with population aging, the well-being of future generations, and the enduring presence of generous benefit packages insured by government. As captured by Neil Howe (personal communication, 1995) of the Concord Coalition, the contemporary divide in the United States along these dimensions finds conservatives favoring dramatic reductions in the role of government in social welfare provision and liberals pressing to tilt social welfare provision more in the direction of young people and away from old people.

The Scope of Age-Based Public Policy

By way of context for the chapters that follow, the following list provides a programmatic and budgetary overview of age-based and age-related policy expenditures in the United State (see Ross 1995; U.S. General Accounting Office 1992; U.S. House of Representatives 1994; U.S. Social Security Administration 1995; Woodside 1996). In an *age-based* program, one of the criteria for eligibility is having attained a specified chronological age; with the exception of the Older Americans Act, there are no programs in which one becomes eligible for benefits simply by virtue of having attained advanced age. *Age-related* programs substantially benefit older people even though the basis for eligibility is independent of chronological age.

- *Means-tested public assistance programs, age-based*

    SSI: Aged people constituted 1.43 million of 6.61 million recipients in June 1996. Of those sixty-five or older receiving benefits, 54.3 percent were seventy-five or older. In 1995, the minimum monthly income ensured by SSI was $446 for older individuals and $687 for older couples. The average monthly SSI payment at the end of 1994 was $243 for an older individual and $617 for an older couple. Total program expenditures for the year ending June 1996 were $28.6 billion.

    Housing: Elderly renters occupied 94 percent of the 138,000 units of Section 202 housing for elderly or handicapped persons in 1988.

- *Means-tested public assistance programs, age-related*

    Food stamps: 17 percent of households receiving food stamps had a member age sixty or older, and 10 percent of recipient families were headed by a woman age sixty or older. Any out-of-pocket medical expense in excess of a $35 deductible was added to deductions from monthly gross income allowed for all recipients in determining benefits for people over age sixty or disabled. In 1990, only an estimated 22 percent of poor elderly persons received food stamps. Early estimates of changes in the food stamp program made as part of 1996 welfare reform legislation were that 1.75 million poor elderly households would lose about 20 percent of their food stamp benefits.

SSI (non-aged-based): In 1994, the elderly constituted 16 percent of people receiving SSI for reason of disability (N = 630,000) and 28 percent of people receiving SSI for reason of blindness (N = 21,000).

Medicaid: Eligibility for Medicaid includes low-income older people who are recipients of SSI (see above), but only 30.2 percent of noninstitutionalized poor elders have Medicaid coverage. Services to people age sixty-five and older accounted for 31 percent of Medicaid expenditures in 1994, or $33.4 billion. Older people made up 11.5 percent of Medicaid beneficiaries. Medicaid accounted for 62 percent of government spending for nursing home care, and such services accounted for nearly two-thirds of Medicaid expenditures on older people. In 1994, the average payment per recipient was $8,364 for persons age sixty-five and older, $7,740 for the disabled, and $1,007 for children.

Housing: Nearly 40 percent of all poor elderly renters benefited from at least one of several federal rental subsidy programs. Elderly people were estimated to occupy between 39 and 45 percent of the nation's 1.3 million public housing units operated by local public housing authorities. Estimates place elderly households at between 30 and 44 percent of all recipients of Section 8 housing certificates and vouchers.

Employment: Low-income people over the age of fifty-five are eligible to participate in the Senior Community Service Employment program (Title V of the Older Americans Act). In 1990, 36,839 people were enrolled. The GAO estimates that some 30,000 of those had incomes below the poverty level, meaning that less than 1 percent of the poor elderly were participating in the program.

• *Summary*

Only 49 percent of the poor elderly population lived in households that received assistance from means-tested federal programs in 1990. In other words, about half of the poor elderly population—1.9 million people—lived in households lacking any form of means-tested federal assistance.

• *Social insurance programs, age-based*

Old Age and Survivors Insurance: The OASI program covered 26.4 million retired workers, 3.1 million spouses and 441,000 children of retired workers, 5.2 million widows and widowers, 1.9 million children and 4,000 parents of deceased workers, and 2,000 people receiving special age-seventy-two benefits. Between 1980 and 1994, program expenditures increased from $105 billion to $279 billion. In 1994, the average monthly benefits for categories of beneficiaries over the age of sixty-five were retired workers ($707), spouses of retired workers ($366), nondisabled widows and widowers ($660), mothers and fathers ($468). In 1994, 71 percent of retired worker, new benefit awards were taken before age sixty-five.

Medicare: In 1994, 32.4 million aged and 4.1 million disabled individuals had protection under Part A, and 31.4 million aged and 3.7 million disabled people were enrolled under Part B; 161,000 people were covered under the End Stage Renal Disease program. The number of aged persons enrolled in Medicare increased from 19.5 million in 1967, to 25.5 million in 1975, to 32.4 million in 1994. Expenditures under Medicare increased from $14.1 billion in 1975 to $162 billion in 1994. Reimbursement per person age sixty-five and sixty-six was $2,851; reimbursement per person age eighty-five and older was $5,337.

- *Social insurance programs, age-related*

  Disability Insurance: In 1994, this program provided benefits to 4 million disabled workers, 271,000 wives and husbands of disabled workers, and 1.35 million children of disabled workers. Average monthly payments were, respectively, $662, $160, and $177. In 1994, 16.4 percent of DI beneficiaries were disabled workers age sixty through sixty-four, down from 24.4 percent in 1988 and 30 percent in 1970.

- *Veterans programs, age-related*

  Because of service in World Wars I and II and the Korean War, expenditures on behalf of military veterans are heavily weighted toward older people. In 1993, service-connected compensation totaling $13.4 billion was paid to 2.2 million disabled veterans and 312,000 survivors. Means-tested veterans' pensions totaling $3.5 billion were paid to war veterans who became permanently and totally disabled from non-service-connected causes and to survivors of war veterans (894,000 people). In 1993, inpatient and outpatient medical and health-related services were provided through the Department of Veterans Affairs to 2.8 million veterans at a cost of $14.8 billion.

Older people and others also benefit from favorable tax provisions that might alternatively have been accomplished through direct expenditures. These so-called tax expenditures are "revenue losses under the

Table 1.2.
Age-Related Tax Expenditure Estimates, 1995

Item	Revenue Loss ($billions)
Today's older population	
Exclusion of Social Security and railroad retirement income	23.1
Exclusion of Medicare Part A benefits	8.0
Exclusion of Medicare Part B benefits	5.1
Additional standard deduction for elderly and blind	1.9
Exclusion of capital gain on sale of residence, persons aged > 55	4.9
Tomorrow's older population	
Net exclusion of pension contributions and earnings	69.5
Keogh plans	3.2
Individual retirement plans	8.4

individual and corporate income tax laws that are attributable to special exclusions, exemptions, or deductions from gross income, or to special credits, preferential rates of tax, or deferrals of tax liability" (U.S. Office of Management and Budget 1979). Tax expenditures apply to a host of individuals and entities and account for a very substantial amount of revenue forgone to (in contrast to expenditure made by) the federal government. Some of the most substantial are age based (specifying ages for eligibility or being tied to programs that do) and age related (providing tax advantages to current workers to encourage them to set aside resources for their retirement). Table 1.2 itemizes the principal tax expenditures related to old people of today and tomorrow.

Conclusion

Public policy based on advanced age has undergone a serious transformation over the last few decades, from "We can't do enough" to "Have we done too much?" Controversies around age seem certain to mount in the years ahead. Addressing the needs of old people will inevitably be an expensive proposition; the key question will be how to allocate costs among older individuals, their families, community agencies, the proprietary sector, and government. Policy discussions will increasingly be affected by ethical dilemmas centering on health care rationing, the right (or obligation) to die, and the right (or obligation) to work. Generational tensions may mount, depending on whether the debate centers on inequities between generations or reciprocity among generations.

Most broadly, the future of age-based policy will be fundamentally caught up in discussions about the role and obligations of government in American life. Those who would reduce the federal government's presence cannot avoid taking on policies for old people because that is where so much of federal domestic expenditures lies. Those who favor renewed federal attention for old people must first see this larger debate, for it will shape and constrain what happens to populations and problems of all sorts. A strategy favored by many would be to extend federal protection to persons who are not yet old but whose old age would be of much higher quality by virtue of having been better served earlier in life, for in addressing the needs of emerging generations, and especially the younger members of those generations, investment is also being made in the betterment of future cohorts of old people.

References

Ball, R. 1985. Commencement Address, University of Maryland–Baltimore County, Catonsville, Md.

Brody, S. 1987. Strategic Planning: The Catastrophic Approach. *Gerontologist* 27:131–38.

Brown, M. 1988. Remaking the Welfare State: A Comparative Perspective. In M. Brown, ed., *Remaking the Welfare State: Retrenchment and Social Policy in America and Europe*. Philadelphia: Temple University Press.

Burke, V., and V. Burke. 1974. *Nixon's Good Deed*. New York: Columbia University Press.

Dolinsky, A., and I. Rosenwaike. 1988. The Role of Demographic Factors in the Institutionalization of the Elderly. *Research on Aging* 10:235–57.

Esping-Andersen, G. 1990. *The Three Worlds of Welfare Capitalism*. Princeton: Princeton University Press.

Gramlich, E. Forthcoming. Different Approaches for Dealing with Social Security. *Journal of Economic Perspectives*.

Heclo, H. 1974. *Modern Social Politics in Britain and Sweden*. New Haven: Yale University Press.

Hudson, R. 1988. Politics and the New Old. In R. Morris and S. Bass, eds., *Retirement Reconsidered*. New York: Springer.

———. 1996. Social Protection and Services. In R. Binstock and L. George, eds., *Handbook of Aging and the Social Sciences,* 4th ed. San Diego: Academic.

Jones, T. 1996. Strengthening the Current Social Security System. *Public Policy and Aging Report* 7(3): 1, 3–7.

Kasper, J. 1988. *Aging Alone: Profiles and Projections*. New York: Commonwealth Fund.

Kotlikoff, L. 1996. Generational Accounting. *Public Policy and Aging Report* 7(4): 4–6, 17.

Lamm, R., and H. Lamm. 1996. *The Challenge of an Aging Society.* Denver: Center for Public Policy and Contemporary Issues, University of Denver.

LaPlante, M., and K. Miller. 1992. People with Disabilities in Basic Life Activities in the U.S. *Disability Statistics Abstract,* No. 3. San Francisco: Institute for Health and Aging, University of California.

Laslett, P. 1987. The Emergence of the Third Age. *Ageing and Society* 7:133–60.

Leone, R. 1996. America Can Afford to Grow Old. *Public Policy and Aging Report* 7(4): 1, 15–16.

Lowi, T. 1990. Risks and Rights in the History of American Governments. *Daedalus* 119:17–40.

Marmor, T. 1970. *The Politics of Medicare.* Chicago: Aldine.

Moon, M., and J. Mulvey. 1996. *Entitlements and the Elderly.* Washington, D.C.: Urban Institute.

Morris, R., and S. Bass. 1988. Toward a New Paradigm about Work and Age. In R. Morris and S. Bass, eds., *Retirement Reconsidered.* New York: Springer.

Nelson, D. 1982. Alternative Images of Old Age as the Bases for Policy. In B. Neugarten, ed., *Age or Need?* Beverly Hills, Calif.: Sage.

Neugarten, B. 1974. Age Groups in American Society and the Rise of the Young-Old. *Annals* 415:187–98.

Quadagno, J. 1996. Social Security and the Myth of the Entitlement "Crisis." *Gerontologist* 36:391–99.

Quinn, J., and R. Burkhauser. 1990. Work and Retirement. In R. Binstock and L. George, eds., *Handbook of Aging and the Social Sciences,* 3d ed. San Diego: Academic.

Radner, D. 1996. Incomes of the Elderly and Non-Elderly, 1967–92. *Social Security Bulletin* 58:82–97.

Rimlinger, G. 1971. *Welfare Policy and Industrialization in Europe, America, and Russia.* New York: Wiley.

Ross, J. 1995. Means-Tested Programs: An Overview of Problems and Issues. Testimony before the Committee on Agriculture, U.S. House of Representatives, Feb. 7.

Rubinow, A. 1934. *The Quest for Security.* New York: Holt.

Schieber, S. 1996. A New Vision for Social Security. Testimony before the Finance Subcommittee on Social Security and Family Policy, U.S. Senate, Mar. 25.

Schulz, J. 1995. *The Economics of Aging.* Westport, Conn.: Auburn House.

Stockman, D. 1975. The Social Pork Barrel. *Public Interest* 39:3–30.

Thomson, D. 1989. The Welfare State and Generation Conflict: Winners and Losers. In P. Johnson, C. Conrad, and D. Thomson, eds., *Workers and Pensioners.* New York: St. Martin's.

U.S. Bureau of the Census. 1988. *Measuring the Effect of Benefits and Taxes on Income and Poverty, 1986.* Washington, D.C.: Government Printing Office.

————. 1992. *Households, Families, and Children: A Thirty-Year Perspective.* Washington, D.C.: Government Printing Office.

U.S. General Accounting Office. 1992. *Elderly Americans: Health, Housing, and Nutrition Gaps between the Poor and Nonpoor.* Washington, D.C.: Government Printing Office.

U.S. House of Representatives, Committee on Ways and Means. 1994. *Overview of Entitlement Programs.* Washington, D.C.: Government Printing Office.

U.S. Office of Management and Budget. 1979. *Budget of the Government of the United States.* Washington, D.C.: Government Printing Office.

U.S. Social Security Administration. 1995. *Annual Statistical Supplement to the Social Security Bulletin.* Washington, D.C.: Government Printing Office.

Wilensky, H., and C. Lebeaux. 1965. *Industrial Society and Social Welfare.* New York: Free Press.

Woodside, C. 1996. *Personal Responsibility and Work Opportunity Reconciliation Act of 1996: Summary of Provisions.* Washington, D.C.: National Association of Social Workers, Office of Government Relations.

PART I

THE COMPETING BASES FOR POLICY BENEFITS

2

Ethics and Public Policy
A Normative Defense of Age-Based Entitlements

MARTHA HOLSTEIN

A combination of ethical reasoning and political necessity justifies the existence and continuation of Social Security and Medicare as age-segregated rather than age-integrated public policies. The central feature of these two programs—universal access to benefits in the absence of means testing—ought to be preserved for two specifically ethical reasons: strengthening human dignity and recognizing social solidarity. The former value is deeply embedded in American ethical, political, and religious reflection; the latter is a less prominent and often inchoate value but also finds roots in American religious and civic traditions. These two values are mutually dependent: dignity focuses central attention on the individual, but the nurturance of dignity requires personal and public commitments based on a sense of connectedness and common ends.

The endorsement here of age-based public policies is not an unqualified defense of policies, even universal ones, based on chronological age. Rather, the argument is that, at this point in time in U.S. political history, advanced age does meet the moral demands of dignity and solidarity and, in the absence of commitment to some understanding of "citizenship rights" (see Myles, this volume), no other broad-based universal eligibility criterion is to be found in the United States. Because universalism in U.S. social policy is confined largely to old people, only these age-based policies serve notice of what has been accomplished in the United States, the responsibilities the country has assumed through public policy, and the obligations it has to the future and to other populations.

Although many policy analysts, knowingly or not, separate policy and ethics (see Amy 1984), ethical values inevitably infiltrate public policy—how it is made, how it is analyzed, and how it is evaluated. It is impossible, for example, to separate the "facts" that analysts rely on from the "values" they promote or shun. Even cost-benefit analysis, the seemingly most objective and value-free approach to public policy, presumes a hierarchy of values, giving the highest value to efficiency. While currently much in vogue, efficiency is but one ethical value that might undergird policy choices; other prominent ethical nominees include justice (in its several different conceptions), rights, respect, human welfare, and the good of future generations. While no public policy (i.e., a mandated allocational scheme) can fulfill all important ethical values, an ethical analysis can illuminate the choices at stake when policies are under development, when changes are proposed, and when they are evaluated. More fundamentally, an ethical analysis can and should lead to moral conclusions and provide the normative basis for advocating on behalf of one position over another (Momeyer 1990).

Attributing primary moral importance to dignity and social solidarity affirms these to be valued moral goods, which are superior to economic or market values centered on efficiency and which cannot be sacrificed without compelling moral reasons. Take, for example, the difficulties of arguing on the basis of efficiency for home care for frail elders and against nursing home care. If it is not, in all cases, cheaper to care for people with serious disabilities in their own homes, that economic "fact of efficiency" could justify nursing home placement. Surely there are other important values associated with what it means to live a good life that are not so socially indulgent as to break the bank and lose all sight of legitimate efficiency concerns.

The Programs

Social Security and Medicare remain extremely popular public programs despite ongoing efforts to shrink, privatize, or otherwise dismantle them. While there is room for dispute at the margins about their aggregate contributions—for example, around Medicare's almost exclusive focus on acute care—the very popularity of these programs suggests that most people believe their goals are both important and reasonably well met. For example, while expressing some concerns about Medicare's coverage and complexities, older people value the sense of security it provides, its ease of enrollment, and its substantial coverage of high-cost hospital care (Kaiser Family Foundation 1994). More generally, there is broad societal consensus that poverty and ill health in old age are sources of threat that deserve a response (adapted from Baier 1985).

Although both Social Security and Medicare have been modified over the years, their underlying premises of universal coverage, earned benefits, and pooled risk have, until very recently, remained essentially unquestioned. The challenges that these values now face arise from differing interpretations of the numbers (e.g., would lowering Medicare expenditures by some $200 billion of projections under current law over a seven-year period be a "cut," even though expenditures would continue to increase?), of the relationship between these entitlement programs and a balanced federal budget, and of older people themselves (are they legitimate recipients of public benefits or are they selfish consumers of scarce social resources?). The recent assaults on Medicare and Social Security represent direct challenges to the values of dignity and social solidarity, the core ethical substructure of the two programs.

Currently, Medicare and, to a lesser extent, Social Security aim to approximate health care and income benefits available to a relatively well-employed younger person (that is, someone who receives a regular salary or wage and medical benefits) without requiring older people to meet eligibility tests other than that associated with their employment history. This serves the values of dignity and solidarity. Yet arguments continue to build against distributing income and medical care benefits in this manner.

One critique holds that age-based entitlements, in a putatively resource-scarce environment, deprive poor people of all ages of support that might otherwise be available to them and impose on younger people payroll tax burdens that are onerous and inequitable. These concerns are central to generational equity concerns, generating proposals to partially privatize Social Security (add a defined contribution tier to the existing defined benefit tier) and Medicare (transform Medicare into a defined contribution plan and introduce medical savings accounts). A second argument critical of these two programs centers on deficit reduction rather than benefits and costs. In many circles, it is now accepted that bringing the deficit into balance is an impossible task without controlling age-based entitlement spending.

These concerns about distribution and deficit reduction, which have stimulated renewed attention to the age-versus-need debate in social policy circles, should be addressed, yet that would not address the central concern here—that income maintenance and access to medical care in old age should be provided in ways that protect dignity and enhance social solidarity. These are critical social goods that must remain in the forefront of any discussion involving these programs. These moral values ought not to be eclipsed.

Dignity

Essential at all ages, dignity is most threatened in old age, when much in our social environment contributes to its erosion. The importance of dignity escalates when a sense of otherness (de Beauvoir 1972) overcomes the belief that one is a person worthy of respect. Thus, while one can legitimately question whether age is becoming increasingly irrelevant as a "predictor of lifestyle or need," one must still ask if that same irrelevancy holds for dignity and self-respect (Binstock 1994, 726). And while the state and society can give an individual neither dignity nor self-respect, they can provide conditions that either support or discourage its recognition and achievement (Walzer 1983).

As contributory and universal programs, Social Security and Medicare have supported the dignity of their recipients. In *A Theory of Justice*, Rawls (1972) emphasizes the securing of self-respect or self-esteem. People, he argues, "would wish to avoid at almost any cost the social conditions that undermine their self-respect," which is "perhaps the most important of all the primary goods" (440, 396). For Taylor (1989), dignity shapes, and therefore is prior to, our choices, desires, and interests and gives them a strong evaluative component. What we consider our autonomous choices actually rest on some moral vision that is "uncommonly deep, powerful, and universal" (ibid., 4) and helps define who we are. Our choices are thus related to our need to see ourselves as having dignity. Goodin (1982) identifies "moral primitives," for which no further justification is needed; dignity is central. This moral concern is not secondary to "either rational articulations of what an unencumbered human would choose or what utility calculations [e.g., cost-benefit analysis] suggest" (Taylor 1989, 8). Dignity demands a minimum standard of decent treatment for every individual and is "not to be sacrificed for any less weighty considerations" (Goodin 1982, 85).

While there may be a number of arguments about the virtues of charity and the dangers of entitlement, dignity is well supported through entitlements based on work history and age, which at that point in the life cycle are comparable to earning one's salary and receiving benefits by virtue of doing one's job. For example, most working-age individuals have had, at least until recently, health insurance offered as a job-related benefit. Receipt of these benefits was not contingent on their inability to purchase insurance on their own. Nor do they expect to pay higher copayments or deductibles if they happen to be high earners. In fact, quite often the opposite has been the case: benefits for corporate executives have become more bountiful while other employees have faced cutbacks (Meyerson 1996).

Medicare permits continuity of values and expectations available during employment years for people no longer employed. Yet, should the age of eligibility be raised for full Social Security and Medicare benefits, hardships would be created for those forced to take early retirement and who would now have no access to health insurance in the private market (see Moon, this volume). The loss of this sense of continuity—and threatening the equality that Medicare affords old people vis-à-vis working people—could clearly undermine feelings of self-respect and dignity. While not usually phrased this way in the policy debate, this notion of dignity is at the heart of the similarities between Medicare and private insurance and distinguishes both of them from the means-tested Medicaid program. In the latter case, stigma cannot coexist with dignity.

Social Solidarity and Human Interdependence

Age-based entitlements, particularly Social Security, also recall values of social solidarity and human interdependence. In an era that focuses so strongly on individual autonomy, Social Security reminds us, in the language of many folk beliefs, that "I am because we are." Each of us owes a debt to past generations; we would, quite literally, not exist "had not someone and some society taken responsibility for our welfare. . . . If we value our own life at all, then we must value and feel some obligation toward those who made that life possible" (Callahan 1981, 77). Age-based policy recognizes that we are, throughout our lives, linked to others and that we would not have grown to be adults without the help of previous generations (Wolfe 1989). Such ties are a "matter of moral intuition, social common sense, and obligatory notions of reciprocity, part of what once was called civil society" (ibid., 101). Over the course of a life, ties of social obligation and reciprocity are ways to ensure that, for example, we raise the next generation of children to understand the meaning of justice or to know what a promise means (Baier 1994; Elshtain 1995).

Social Security, though framed in terms of a contract, more accurately embodies what are deeply held notions of reciprocity. While relations of social obligation and reciprocity are not always freely chosen, they are required for the continuity of a just society (Baier 1994). The fact that each of us pays into the system and then anticipates receiving benefits through a tacit relationship with generations to follow reinforces the important moral concern with reciprocity. This aspect deserves more attention than it has received. Such bonds are not merely incidental; they are morally honorable and necessary. The privatization of Social Security, seen earlier as a threat to dignity, undermines the tenets of solidarity, as well, by challenging the intergenerational linkages embodied in social security.

Social solidarity is a "necessary condition for the flourishing of the subjective life"; a human being understood holistically is more socially committed, socially shaped, and socially nourished than much recent ethical thinking would have us believe (Anjos 1994, 139). In contemporary American society, there are few public expressions of social solidarity and interdependence. Yet, many of our deepest moral sentiments, supported by research in moral psychology and other domains, reinforce the importance of the social. Without visible expressions of community, we lack the social glue that binds each of us as individuals into a society. Yet, we rarely acknowledge the social goals of Social Security and Medicare and so do not stimulate informed discussion about the losses that might occur if those goals withered.

Practically, Social Security permits the sharing of risks at a time in life when risk is most imminent. Apart from Social Security protections directed at younger persons—notably, survivors' and dependents' benefits—Social Security helps ensure the stability of generations over time by very considerably alleviating the need for younger generations to help finance their parents' retirement. Indeed, the proportion of older persons' income provided by family members has dropped from an estimated 50 percent before the enactment of Social Security to only 2 percent today (Brody 1987).

One need only recall the "family economies" of the late nineteenth and early twentieth centuries (Haber and Gratton 1994) to understand the potentially bruising results that future generations would experience from increased family responsibility. For the older generation, Social Security lessens fears about being a burden on their children and, for some, facilitates continued contributions to successor generations. In this way, it encourages the ongoing recognition and practice of reciprocal and interdependent relationships while mitigating the troubling aspects of asymmetrical relationships that develop as parents need more from their children.

Social Security can also make a practical contribution to maintaining ties of interdependency and solidarity. The normative life course, which Social Security helps create and sustain, frees up a number of individuals, often in relatively good health, to contribute to society in ways often unavailable to younger working parents of families. We might, of course, achieve the same ends if benefits were needs based, but it would be less likely for two reasons. First, the sense of security that comes with age-based entitlements is liberating and can encourage the person to pursue socially constructive interests. Second, there is the risk—very pertinent today in the light of recent reforms to the Aid to Families with Dependent Children program—that means testing will impose work requirements on healthy people without concern for the number or quality of jobs available. In this way, the possibilities of contributing to the social good through alternative activities would be reduced.

Alternative Frameworks

It is not impossible, though very unlikely, that means-tested programs could ensure the same relative security now available through Medicare and Social Security. It is even less likely, however, that they could support the two moral values this chapter holds as central. Both U.S. history and the contemporary political scene mitigate against this possibility. Benefits offered as age-based entitlements do not require explicitly determined needs that others have the power to define (Elshtain 1995).

Means testing would require older people, at a time when they may already have lost much of what is valued in American society, to "prove" their worthiness to gatekeepers of resources. They would have to do so in the face of many competing priorities for public resources in a period of tough parsimony—or what some call tough love. There are also significant racial and gender dimensions to consider. Those who will be in the competitive pool are far more likely to be women, especially women of color. This in itself presents another significant problem of justice. In the late nineteenth century, the English researcher Charles Booth conducted an extensive study of poverty. He found that "there is no parallel in feeling between the taking of a sum of money to which a man is legally entitled and the suing *in forma-pauperis* for a benefit that might be granted or postponed or withheld, and the granting of which must, in the public interest, be protected by preliminary suspicion and searching inquiry" (quoted in Goodin 1985, 37–38).

Moreover, we could not ensure that future political leaders would not hold lower-income older people "accountable" for their low incomes. Blame, not unfamiliar on the U.S. political landscape, is inherently antithetical to dignity and solidarity. It is better, therefore, that some get more than they need than that the many be left with an uncertain future when they have scarce opportunity to improve their situation. The tax system provides the most equitable vehicle to moderate even this outcome. Moreover, "it is arguable that more poor elderly have been helped by the relative invulnerability of age-based programs than would have been helped had programs been more narrowly targeted to the poor" (Daniels 1988, 10). The generational equity debate reinforces this insight. While offering the vision of "greedy geezers," clearly inimical to any notions of dignity or social solidarity, those promoting that view have proposed little to attend to the needs of either poor children or vulnerable elders. Instead, in delegitimating the deservingness of older people, that debate served as the first act of the rescue drama now unfolding, currently featuring the Concord Coalition and the Third Millennium.

It is not only the immediate debate that urges wariness with needs-based programs. Except perhaps in the colonial period, when communities took care of their own with minimum fuss, this country's public and private welfare programs have been both niggardly and judgmental. In the nineteenth and early twentieth centuries, even the aged, as a category of the deserving poor, had few options but the almshouse if their families could not care for them (Haber and Gratton 1994; Holstein and Cole 1996). The almshouse supported neither dignity nor solidarity. Nor was it ever designed to provide income or anything but the most modest medical care.

It is also well to remember that losses often accumulate in old age. New images of "successful" or "productive" aging cannot foreclose this reality for large numbers of older people. The death of a spouse or even a child, illness, and disability give the older person few chances to recoup. Savings are quickly consumed and emotional reserves exhausted. Yet it would be at this very time that the older person would have to prove worthy of public support if programs were means tested. Bracketing the practical problems of determining levels and kinds of support, one can easily see the assault on dignity that would result. Simultaneously, when individuals are at their weakest, the necessity for social solidarity is the strongest. Needs-based programs cannot respond to this requirement.

Once the goals of Social Security and Medicare are extended to include the moral values of dignity and social solidarity, arguments based on the utilitarian criteria of efficiency and effectiveness become difficult to support. Such arguments rarely include these nonquantifiable moral values. Without addressing the wide-ranging critique of such thinking (see Williams and Sen 1982), one can say that it ignores much of what moral psychology has learned about what humans value and how these values support qualitative distinctions of worth (Taylor 1989). Arguments based solely on utilitarian criteria cannot sustain a broad democratic ethos in which ties of relationship are central and in which the notion of citizenship means active participation in the good of the community. Efficiency/effectiveness arguments thus obscure important social values. Efficiency is but one among many values that ought to count in deciding how to respond to human need. Seemingly quantifiable, efficiency "purges moral analysis of all of its difficult—and essential—characteristics" (Amy 1984, 587). Its singularity means that choices among competing ethical values do not even appear as problematic.

Conclusion

While Social Security and Medicare cannot alone support a wavering democratic ethos, they serve as reminders that ties of social obligation (even if not specifically chosen) and mutual interdependence are part of what it means to be human. Moreover, they contribute to the provision of social goods that most of us view as primary. Of course, one might suggest that, since these goods are so highly valued, they be made available to all Americans. And if our social accounting considered all social welfare costs rather than only direct costs, we might discover the resources necessary to provide these goods more broadly. However, given the unlikeliness of such a scenario, it makes no sense to take away from old people what would be desirable for all to have.

Acknowledgments

The author is appreciative of the thoughtful questions raised by David Mccurdy, Larry Greenfield, W. Patrick Hill, and Deb Harris-Abbott, colleagues at the Park Ridge Center.

References

Amy, D. 1984. Why Policy Analysis and Ethics Are Incompatible. *Journal of Policy Analysis and Management* 3:573–91.

Anjos, M. 1994. Bioethics in a Liberationist Key. In E. Dubose, R. Hamel, and L. O'Connell, eds., *A Matter of Principles? Ferment in U.S. Bioethics.* Valley Forge, Penn.: Trinity Press International.

Baier, A. 1985. *Postures of the Mind.* Minneapolis: University of Minnesota Press.

———. 1994. *Moral Prejudices: Essays on Ethics.* Cambridge: Harvard University Press.

Binstock, R. 1994. Changing Criteria in Old-Age Programs: The Introduction of Economic Status and Need. *Gerontologist* 34:726–30.

Brody, S. 1987. Strategic Planning: The Catastrophic Approach. *Gerontologist* 27:131–38.

Callahan, D. 1981. What Obligations Do We Have to Future Generations? In E. Partridge, ed., *Responsibilities to Future Generations Environmental Ethics.* Buffalo, N.Y.: Prometheus.

Daniels, N. 1988. *Am I My Parent's Keeper?* New York: Oxford University Press.

de Beauvoir, S. 1972. *The Coming of Age.* New York: Putnam.

Elshtain, J. 1995. *Democracy on Trial.* New York: Basic Books.

Goodin, R. 1982. *Political Theory and Public Policy.* Chicago: University of Chicago Press.

———. 1985. Self-Reliance versus the Welfare State. *Journal of Social Policy* 14:25–47.

Haber, C., and B. Gratton. 1994. *Old Age and the Search for Security.* Bloomington: University of Indiana Press.

Holstein, M., and T. Cole. 1996. The History of Long-Term Care in America. In R. Binstock, L. Cluff, and O. von Mering, eds., *The Future of Long-Term Care.* Baltimore: Johns Hopkins University Press.

Kaiser Family Foundation. 1994. Seniors Have Mixed Emotions about Medicare. News Release, Oct. 4.

Meyerson, A. 1996. Executives Are Cradled while Medical Benefits Are Cut for Rank and File. *New York Times,* Mar. 17.

Momeyer, R. 1990. Philosophers and the Public Policy Process: Inside, Outside, or Nowhere at All. *Journal of Medicine and Philosophy* 15:391–409.

Rawls, J. 1972. *A Theory of Justice.* Cambridge: Harvard University Press.

Taylor, C. 1989. *Sources of the Self.* Cambridge: Harvard University Press.

Walzer, M. 1983. *Spheres of Justice: A Defense of Pluralism and Equality.* New York: Basic Books.

Williams, B., and A. Sen. 1982. *Utilitarianism and Beyond.* Cambridge: Cambridge University Press.

Wolfe, A. 1989. *Whose Keeper? Social Science and Moral Obligation.* Berkeley: University of California Press.

3

Why the Graying of the Welfare State Threatens to Flatten the American Dream—or Worse

NEIL HOWE

Despite overwhelming evidence that the cost of major senior benefit programs is due to explode over the next half-century, the notion persists that they are sustainable without major cost cuts. Although tax rates may rise, this argument runs, a growing economy will still allow workers to enjoy steady gains in real after-tax earnings. However, an examination of the likely future fiscal and tax impact of three major senior programs—Social Security, Medicare, and Medicaid for people age sixty-five and older—demonstrates that this argument is clearly wrong. Projections based on a model that incorporates all of the official assumptions used by the Social Security Administration and the Health Care Financing Administration in calculating the growth of the three programs show that, absent major reform, the graying of the welfare state is likely to have catastrophic consequences for the after-tax living standards of most working-age Americans (scenarios ii and iii, in U.S. Federal Old-Age and Survivors Insurance 1994). In particular, depending on the scenario employed, earnings per U.S. worker will remain unchanged between 1995 and 2040 or could fall—in real terms—as much as 59 percent. Moreover, governmental spending as a percentage of the GNP will grow from today's 34.4 percent to as much as 55 percent by 2040.

The practical bottom line of this analysis speaks for itself. America's political leaders cannot continue in good faith to advocate balanced budgets, tax cuts, and leaner government—to say nothing of defending the long-term viability of the American dream—without also talking about major, structural reforms in "untouchable" senior entitlements. Everything must be on the table.

The Unpleasant Facts

In 1994, the American public was bombarded by a spate of official warnings about the crushing public cost that will accompany the rapid aging of the U.S. population early in the twenty-first century. Some examples:

• In April 1994, the Social Security trustees issued an annual report announcing that their combined cash-benefit trust funds would all go belly up in 2029—seven years earlier than they had reported in 1993 and nineteen years earlier than they had reported in 1988 (U.S. Federal Old-Age and Survivors Insurance 1994).

• In August 1994, a bipartisan presidential commission agreed by a thirty-to-one vote that "the government must act now" to prevent just five benefit programs (Social Security, Medicare, Medicaid, and federal civilian and military pensions) from consuming total federal revenues by the year 2030 (U.S. Bipartisan Commission 1994).

• In September 1994, the U.S. Congressional Budget Office (1994) confirmed that over the following decade entitlements would grow from roughly half to two-thirds of all federal spending. "The aging of the baby-boom generation," added the CBO, "will continue to drive that share higher over succeeding decades."

• And in October 1994, Alice Rivlin, the director of the Office of Management and Budget, leaked a budget options memo that illustrated how annual budget deficits would soar above $4.1 trillion by 2030 under current tax and spending policies.

By now, the public has little problem comprehending the overall arithmetic of the situation. It is widely understood that retirement, disability, and (especially) health benefits outlays are already among the fastest-growing categories of governmental spending.

Asked about the growing numerical imbalance of retirees to workers in the Social Security System, 64 percent of American adults say it is a "very serious" problem; 29 percent say it is "somewhat serious."

Asked the same question about the impact of runaway health care costs on the survival of Medicare, 78 percent say it is "very serious"; 19 percent say it is "somewhat serious." To either question, only about 5 percent say "not too serious," "not at all a problem," or "don't know" (Matthew Greenwald 1994). According to a 1994 *New York Times*/CBS News poll, 58 percent of adults now think that "the next generation's future will be worse than life today"; only 18 percent think it will be better. What is more, baby boomers realize they are in line to take the hit: 85 percent of boomers agree that "government has made financial promises to my generation that it will not be able to keep" (Merrill Lynch 1994).

Many say they are ready to face up. Although Americans are understandably ambivalent about cutting benefits that flow to just over half of all U.S. households, neither have they become irredeemable entitlement addicts. Asked about "the financial problems of the Social Security and Medicare systems," 78 percent of all adults (83% of everyone under age fifty) agree that the problems are "so severe that major reforms are needed now" in both programs. A large and growing majority favors imposing a strict means test on major federal entitlement programs (Matthew Greenwald 1994).

Why Politicians Do Not Act

But although voters are rousing themselves, most of our national political leaders are still running for cover. Even in the wake of the stunning anti-big-government message from voters in November 1994, members of Congress in both parties quickly lined up to declare that the vast senior share of the federal budget remains undiscussable. Many remain convinced that the "age wave" forecasts are overblown, that the public talks bolder than it walks, and that in the end the United States will be able to muddle through without "tough choices" or "major reforms." Hence their claim that economizers need only cut domestic discretionary programs—and that the political risks of attempting surgery on senior benefits far outweigh the risks of doing nothing.

To the extent that there is a rational justification for this position, the logic tends to gravitate around three propositions: one, the assumptions underlying the official benefit forecasts are too pessimistic; two, the cost explosion in health care benefits will recede as a result of relatively painless "comprehensive" reforms; or three, if one and two do not explain things away, a tolerable tax hike can be levied on future workers to fund whatever health and cash benefit growth remains.

The first proposition, alas, is not an argument at all, but an attitude. Many legislators chafe at the political inexpedience of rules that force them to take long-term costs into account. But no one presses a comprehensive case that the official "intermediate cost" economic and demographic scenario—offered by the Social Security trustees as their "best estimate"—is overly pessimistic. The reason is simple: for most of the important variables, these assumptions are decidedly more optimistic than actual U.S. experience over the past quarter of a century. Yes, one does hear the occasional exclamation about recent trends in immigration or the birthrate. But all this is small potatoes at best, especially since there has been no actuarially favorable change in trends in labor productivity or longevity—the two assumptions that totally dominate the cost outcome well past the year 2040. That means the intermediate cost projection had better be taken seriously.

What about health care? Everyone agrees that health care benefits are a major part of the projection equation, constituting much of the expected growth in total benefits. Almost everyone agrees that policy changes could do something to control that growth. What is doubtful, however, is whether either political party is likely to champion any change that might make a real difference. On the left, there is much tough talk about draconian "cost containment," but few members have ever identified a single benefit, service, or subsidy in Medicare or Medicaid that ought to be cut. To the contrary, health reforms offered by liberals point toward vast cost increases beyond current projections—including a wider safety net for low-income families and new benefits for older people covering prescription drugs and at-home and long-term care. Conservatives are not as tied to benefit expansion, but neither have they shown much interest in means testing or rationing publicly funded health services. The outlook for health care spending is made even bleaker by another little-known fact: the official long-term projections for Medicare and Medicaid already assume that a vigorous program of cost control will commence early in the next century.

Given the weakness of the first and second propositions, a lot rides on the third: just raise taxes and pray that they do not have to be raised too much. At the very least, the prevailing inertia on entitlement makes this possibility of serious interest to all Americans. What

Table 3.1.
Annual Cost of Social Security and Medicare (Parts A and B) as a Percentage
of Workers' Taxable Payroll

Calendar Year	Intermediate-Cost Projection	High-Cost Projection
1993	16.5	16.5
2010	21.4	26.7
2025	30.5	43.0

Source: U.S. Federal Old-Age and Survivors Insurance (1994).

happens to taxes if we leave all currently legislated benefit provisions
on autopilot? Specifically, how high will taxes rise on future workers?

Table 3.1 offers a suggestive, if partial, answer to this question. It
shows the projected future cost of Social Security and Medicare as a
percentage of the FICA-taxable wages of all U.S. workers covered by
the programs. Two official projections (intermediate cost and high
cost) are tabulated.

What Happens to After-Tax Earnings?

Few politicians actually advocate burdening future workers with costs
of this magnitude. When forced to confront the issue, most voters'
first inclination is to declare that such tax hikes would be unfair, if not
unthinkable. Defenders of the entitlement status quo, however, have
long labored to change the terms of the debate and to make the unthinkable seem really pretty decent after all. Even if the tax rate of future worker earnings must ultimately climb, they argue, real pretax
earnings will still grow swiftly enough to allow future workers to
enjoy a steady rise in real after-tax pay. In other words, they claim, tomorrow's workers will be so well off that they can afford to fork over
a larger share of their income to government and still be a lot better
off than today's workers.

The importance of this claim to the case against cost cutting can
hardly be overemphasized. If true, it means that the current policy
drift is less alarming than is portrayed by the reformers. Even if the official projections are right on the mark, in the end our kids can easily
afford to take up the slack. If true, it also strengthens other arguments
that tend to legitimize today's institutional arrangements. For example,
the often-cited "life cycle" defense of Social Security and Medicare
(which reassures the rising generation that even if they now feel
fleeced by the old, they will someday be able to fleece a new rising

generation in their turn) depends critically on the programs' permanence. Most people would probably doubt this permanence if the programs did not allow workers to enjoy a significant growth rate in after-tax living standards.

Small wonder that the claim about how our kids will be better off anyway (so why worry) crops up so often. "Don't shed too many tears for generations who will be working and retiring in the 21st century," said Nobel Prize-winning economist James Tobin. "They will be living higher than we did and do" (Tobin 1987).

According to the former Social Security Administration commissioner Robert Ball, the extra taxes necessary to fund Social Security in the next century are "not trivial, but easily supportable" by future workers—and "not really a big deal." He then goes on to calculate that the extra taxes needed by 2025 would only "offset about 8 percent of the growth in earnings projected between now and then" ("Social Security: Is It Affordable?" *Washington Post,* February 15, 1994).

Henry Aaron, the Brookings Institution's economic studies director, contends that "even if we do nothing to change present policies, modest economic growth will produce increases in consumption that dwarf the added cost of caring for the Baby Boom Generation in retirement" (1988). One might expect that a claim so often repeated would be carefully researched. Surprisingly, this not the case. Most often, the claim comes with no supporting evidence; when it does, the calculations are out of date, look at only cash benefits, or fail to account for the total tax burden on earnings.

So, is the claim, in fact, true? A computerized study of the government's own long-term projections reveals that it almost certainly is not. An analysis of the official intermediate-cost and high-cost scenarios shows that raising taxes to cover the cost growth of three major programs—Social Security, Medicare, and Medicaid benefits to seniors—will have a devastating impact on future after-tax wage growth. These scenarios indicate that, between now and about the year 2040, real after-tax earnings will stagnate at best. Quite possibly (again, assuming no major reform), they will plunge steeply.

Incomes Model and Findings

These conclusions are derived from a computer model of future after-tax earnings that are consistent with the official Social Security Administration (SSA) and Health Care Financing Administration

(HCFA), scenarios ii and iii, as published in their 1994 annual trustees' reports. The model isolates the historical and projected growth of Social Security, Medicare, and Medicaid benefits received by people age sixty-five and older.

To derive after-tax earnings continuously into the future, certain assumptions were necessary in addition to those provided by SSA and HCFA (see Howe 1994). The major ones are:

• When the Old Age, Survivors, and Disability Insurance (OASDI) or Hospital Insurance trust funds go bust, they immediately switch over to pay-as-you-go financing.

• All other governmental spending besides Social Security, Medicare, and Medicaid for older people will continue to rise at the same rate as the GDP.

• Between 1995 and 2010, the net public sector budget will move to balance and then stay balanced, proportionally adjusting all types of public revenues as necessary.

• The incidence of total taxation on workers follows plausible theory.

The major findings of my model are the following. (All per-worker figures are translated into constant 1993 dollars.)

• Under the intermediate-cost projection (scenario ii), real after-tax earnings per U.S. worker will remain virtually unchanged between 1995 and 2040. In 1995, after-tax earnings will amount to $19,221. By 2040, they will reach $19,346—less than 1 percent total growth over nearly half a century.

• Under the high-cost projection (scenario iii), real after-tax earnings per U.S. worker will decline 59 percent between 1995 and 2040. In 1995, they will amount to $19,000. By 2040, they will fall to $7,821. Incredibly, this would be a much faster annual rate of decline than the annual rate at which after-tax earnings rose between 1951 and 1970.

• Runaway health care benefits are clearly not the only force behind the rising tax take on worker pay. Under scenario ii, fully 62 percent of the pretax earnings growth between 1995 and 2040 will be wiped out by general government, Social Security, and budget balance. (Medicare will take another 27%, and Medicaid for older people 10%.) Under scenario iii, remarkably, 95 percent of pretax earnings growth will be wiped out by general government, Social Security, and budget balance alone.

• The grim after-tax earnings trends are clearly not the result of pessimistic economic assumptions. Quite the opposite: the optimism of the most important economic assumption—pretax earnings—is very visible. From the early 1970s to the early 1990s, pretax earnings hardly grew at all—in fact, by no more than 0.2 percent annually, no matter which end year you choose. Even during the much vaunted 1979-89 decade, pretax earnings grew by only 0.4 percent annually. Yet from 1995 to 2040, pretax earnings are expected to accelerate to an average of 1.0 percent annually under scenario ii and 0.5 percent annually under scenario iii.

• Trust fund financing mechanisms make little difference in the magnitude or timing of the cost burden on workers.

• Under scenario ii, total governmental benefit spending will rise by nearly 10 percentage points of GDP by 2040. In 1995, benefits will amount to 14.0 percent of GDP; by 2040, 23.5 percent of GDP, nearly what the entire federal government spends today. Meanwhile, total governmental spending will rise from 34.4 to 43.9 percent of GDP.

• Under scenario iii, total governmental benefit spending will rise by nearly 20 percentage points of GDP by 2040. In 1995, benefits will amount to 14.0 percent of GDP; by 2040, 34.1 percent of GDP, roughly what all levels of government spend today. Meanwhile, total governmental spending will rise from 34.4 to 54.5 percent of GDP.

• Under both scenarios, the total tax rate on worker compensation grows steadily. From 41 percent in 1994, it climbs to 57 percent by 2040 under scenario ii and to 69 percent by 2040 under scenario iii.

Conclusion

The foregoing analysis suggests that, absent major reform, the graying of the welfare state is likely to have catastrophic consequences for the after-tax living standards of most working-age Americans.

It has long been known that current-law spending from major entitlement programs is projected to grow considerably faster than our economy under all of the official scenarios. If budgets must be balanced at some point in the future, these scenarios imply an even steeper growth in total tax revenues as a share of GDP and in total tax rates on most definitions of income. Some observers maintain, however, that higher cost as a share of GDP or payroll does not rule out a comfortable growth rate in real after-tax earnings. We show that it does. According to the official best estimate scenario of the Social Security and Medicare trustees, real after-tax earnings will remain entirely stagnant over the next half-century. According to a more prudent scenario, which better reflects recent history, after-tax earnings will decline drastically over the next half-century.

Few Americans would willingly or knowingly embrace either of these visions of the future. For defenders of the entitlement status quo, then, the challenge is not so much to defend the results described here as to question the assumptions that lead to them. But there really is not much opening for direct rebuttal. The most critical assumptions, after all, are embodied in the official economic and demographic scenarios. And while it is easy to imagine a brighter future than scenarios ii or iii, it would be difficult to argue that we should count on such a brighter future on the basis of past experience.

Yes, touching the untouchables is politically dangerous. Any leader who brings up the subject of Social Security or health care for elderly people had better be ready to discuss such gut-level issues as early retirement, "spending down" for Medicaid, the function of the extended family, second liver transplants versus student loans, Lee Iacocca's Social Security check, who should care for other people's wayward children, and how to balance the rightful claims of the young and the old on our public fisc. From there, the discussion moves inevitably toward programmatic options: raising the retirement age, means testing, or prospective capitated health care budgeting. All of these are issues that force most Americans to rethink their own ideals and institutions.

On the other hand, leaving the untouchables alone is also dangerous. Much of the U.S. electorate is convinced that the government has played some enormous scam with their future that no one is willing to talk about. And if the leaders in power do not solve this problem by the time the bills come due, the electorate will surely engage in some heavy retribution—not against who did speak up, but against who did not. Indeed, the willingness of either party to pay attention to these issues is probably an excellent indication of whether that party has any serious intention of governing the nation for long.

References

Aaron, H. 1988. Proceedings of "Children at Risk: Who Will Support Our Aging Society?" Conference sponsored by Americans for Generational Equity and Center for Public Policy and Contemporary Issues, Denver, Colo., May 13.

Howe, N. 1994. *Why the Graying of the Welfare State Threatens to Flatten the American Dream—Or Worse.* Policy Paper 10. Washington, D.C.: National Taxpayers Union.

Matthew Greenwald and Associates, Inc. 1994. *Entitlement Survey.* Washington, D.C.: Congressional Institute for the Future and the National Taxpayers Union Foundation.

Merrill Lynch and Co., Inc. 1994. *Saving the American Dream: An Economic and Public Opinion Study.* New York.

Tobin, J. 1987. An Exchange on Social Security. *New Republic,* May 18, 22.

U.S. Bipartisan Commission on Entitlement and Tax Reform. 1994. *Interim Report to the President.* Washington, D.C.: Government Printing Office.

U.S. Congressional Budget Office. 1994. *Reducing Entitlement Spending.* Washington, D.C.: Government Printing Office.

U.S. Federal Old-Age and Survivors Insurance and Disability Trust Funds, Board of Trustees. 1994. *1994 Annual Report of the Board of Trustees of the Federal Old-Age and Survivors Insurance and Disability Trust Funds.* Washington, D.C.: Government Printing Office.

4

Neither Rights nor Contracts
The New Means Testing in U.S. Aging Policy

JOHN MYLES

In a remarkable essay first presented at Cambridge in 1949 (see Marshall 1964), the British sociologist T. H. Marshall pointed out that the history of Western capitalist democracies has been inextricably linked to the development of citizenship—rights and entitlements that attach to people by virtue of membership in a national community rather than to their property, status, or market capacity. Over a period of some 250 years, these universal principles extended from civil rights (the right to justice, freedom of speech and faith, the right to conclude contracts) to political rights (the right to participate in the exercise of political power, including the right to vote and the right to hold public office) to social rights (the right to a modicum of economic welfare according to the standards prevailing in society).

As a matter of principle (though clearly not always in practice), the United States has since its founding formally adhered to the tenets of civil and political rights. Adherence to principles associated with social rights has, however, been much more limited. In this chapter's first section, these limits are seen in the U.S.'s widespread failure to impose national standards for social welfare provision and in its limiting the values underpinning such programs to those associated with contract (Social Security) and charity (public assistance). The second section finds that the current and prospective problems associated with social welfare for old people lie not in social welfare policy but in the failings of the private market. Future cohorts of elders have good reason to be worried but not for the reasons found in much contemporary debate. I conclude from this analysis that contemporary pressures on aging programs in the United States are only secondarily a question of resources and expenditures. More fundamental is the absence of rights (which cannot be violated), a weakening of contracts (which always can be rewritten), and through the mechanism of federalism, even an attack on charity (which can always be withheld).

Universality and Social Policy in the United States

In the modern era, universality has been applied to social policy in three different ways. First, it is used to identify all social programs that are regulated on the basis of a single set of national standards. In the United States, Old Age, Survivors, and Disability Insurance (OASDI) and Supplemental Security Income (SSI) programs meet this standard, but many other programs—unemployment insurance and Aid to Families with Dependent Children (AFDC)—do not.

Second, universality can refer to social programs available to all citizens independent of either need (the principal eligibility criterion for public assistance) or participation in the labor market (the principal eligibility criterion for social insurance). Unlike some other countries in which national health insurance and family allowances are widespread, virtually no such programs exist in the United States. Medicare is an approximation, but its being largely confined to old persons and its level of deductibles and copayments make it unusual in international comparison. (Ironically, in its early promoting of universal public education, the United States was a nineteenth-century leader in the extension of social citizenship. That most Americans would not categorize public education as "social welfare" lessens the irony considerably.)

A third use of universality with major application to the United States is found in the direct comparison between social insurance and public assistance programs. The former can be said to be universal in the sense of being inclusive of all those who are in the labor force; Social Security is universal, if you will, for the citizen-worker.

In recent years, debates about all three meanings of *universality* have been in play. The issue of national standards has surfaced in the context of Republican proposals to return welfare to the states in the form of block grants to fund Medicaid and AFDC, further decentralizing an already decentralized system. Citizenship issues emerged as part of the debate over the Clinton effort to reform health insurance. And the "universality" of social insurance has surfaced in the context of proposals such as those from the Concord Coalition (Peterson 1993) to restrict benefit eligibility for programs like OASI to families with moderate and low incomes. Each of these meanings of universality bears on current debates about—and the future status of—the elderly and age-based programs. I consider each in turn.

The Case for National Standards

Historically, the establishment of national standards in education, health care, or social policy had more to do with the activities of nation building than with concerns with program equity and efficiency. For national elites, the capacity to mobilize citizens—whether for warfare or welfare—depended greatly on the creation of a national identity buttressed by a common language and loyalties broader than those extending only to local and regional identity.

In many jurisdictions, however, religious, ethnic, and linguistic differences were overcome only by accommodating differences and striking bargains that left significant control in the hands of regional or local elites. The U.S. Constitution was a compromise among colonial elites from regionally distinct economies and societies that were divided, most notably, by the existence of a slave labor system in the South. The result was the creation of a highly decentralized system of government that left considerable jurisdiction in the hands of the states.

Divided jurisdiction—federalism—and the absence of national standards continue to be defining features of the U.S. welfare state. In the original Social Security Act, Old Age Insurance was the only program established that was not a joint program of both the federal government and the states. Considerable movement toward nationalization occurred in the 1960s and 1970s through the establishment of Medicare, the food stamp program, Supplemental Security Income, and the earned-income tax credit. Current discourse, of course, underscores the powerful momentum pushing in the direction of devolution—a return of power to the states.

Both historical experience and considerable theory point to the differences to be expected between local and national programs. In the 1950s, Tiebout (1956) made the case against national standards by arguing that competition among jurisdictions and "jurisdiction shopping" by individuals could operate like any other competitive market and maximize utility among citizens. As Osberg (1992) observes, in contemporary public finance the Tiebout model is generally held up as a straw man with limited general relevance. Where labor is mobile across jurisdictions (as among U.S. states), the production of public goods—especially redistributive policies—tends to be suboptimal, as state and local governments engage in a "race toward the bottom." In the absence of national standards, Peterson and Rom (1988) conclude, state and local governments in a federal system will tend to provide less income distribution than would a national government. Each state government acts as if it prefers that welfare services be provided by other governments and as if it fears that generous benefits will make it attractive to poor people. The pressure for downward harmonization in social benefits has been especially noticeable since the 1970s in AFDC and unemployment insurance. Only jurisdictions that are relatively immune to migration flows because of language (Quebec) or isolated from national labor markets (Oregon, Hawaii) have had the degrees of freedom to experiment with progressive policy reforms at the local level (Skocpol 1992).

One need not be an advocate of greater equality or more redistribution to be concerned with problems created by the race for the bottom created by divided jurisdiction. Keeping state taxes low not only attracts migrants and investors but also repels them. Decisions to migrate and invest reflect the quality of public services (education, health care) available to workers and the quality of labor (educated and healthy) available to employers. In more formal terms, both allocative and dynamic efficiency are impeded when the migration decisions of labor and capital are distorted by variations in public services and benefits. As Osberg (1992, 10) writes: "If the mobility decisions of a significant fraction of the population were to be substantially influenced by differences in the quality of a particular government service, the social cost would be both the excess of migration of those who migrate to take advantage of the service and the excess immobility of those who refuse to move to better jobs because of poorer services elsewhere."

The most relevant application of these observations to older Americans is found in the wide variations in Medicaid provision for long-term care. The decentralized character of Medicaid is part of the reason for the suboptimal quality and quantity of long-term care services in the United States. Decision makers in New York must take into account the return migration potential of very sick elderly people in Florida that could be triggered by a liberalization of New York's Medicaid long-term care provisions. The complete off-loading of Medicaid to the states, as found in proposals recently pending in Washington—especially in the absence of meaningful maintenance-of-effort strictures—can only exacerbate outcomes of this kind.

Universality, Citizenship, and Social Insurance

As Fraser and Gordon (1992) observe, the language of "social citizenship" and "social rights" as understood in European traditions is largely absent from American political discourse. In contrast, the United States does have a richly elaborated discourse of "civil citizenship" that deals with "individual liberties" and "freedom of speech." They write that "U.S. thinking about social provision has been shaped largely by images drawn from civil citizenship, especially images of contract. The result has been to focus on two rather extreme forms of human relationship: discrete contractual exchange of equivalents, juxtaposed against unreciprocated, unilateral charity" (47).

The basic division in which the contract-charity distinction is expressed is between contributory programs such as Social Security, which become "entitlements," and public assistance, in which beneficiaries "get something for nothing" (charity). The relative absence of a discourse of social citizenship and social rights in American life means that debates over social policy inevitably become framed in terms of (contractual) entitlements (Is it really the case that retirees are just getting back what they paid in to Social Security?) or charity (Are these beneficiaries really deserving of our largesse?).

The exception to this generalization is "free" public education at the primary and secondary levels. Indeed, I have found that students in my undergraduate courses become quite upset with proposals to adopt a voucher system, which would subsidize families who send their children to private schools. There is something inherently offensive to the American sense of citizenship in notions that treat primary and secondary education in anything but a universalistic fashion. (President Clinton sought to invoke this social citizenship ethos during the great national health care debate—and failed.) In the area of income transfers, however, there is no tradition of universal benefits or social rights.

In contrast, the concept of universality in the third sense introduced earlier—the inclusion of all workers—bears directly on current
American debates to means-test Social Security, the country's major
social insurance program. As Peterson (1993), one of the main proponents of this idea, puts it, Why should the government be sending out
Social Security checks to wealthy retired investment bankers such as
himself? Means testing is, in this instance, taxing back benefits at an
accelerating rate as incomes rise above $35,000 or $40,000 per year.

Means-testing Social Security might achieve several different objectives. It would make more revenues available to support programs
(such as the earned-income tax credit) for younger families with low
incomes. It is also a partial privatization of the American pension system in that a means test for Social Security represents a supertax on
the social but not the private incomes (investments, pensions) of
elderly people. Through a means test for the affluent, the government
is essentially getting out of the business of selling pension insurance to
high-income earners. Presumably, high-income earners will begin to
purchase more retirement insurance in the private market. There is a
paradox here in that, under current tax law, contributions and earnings in retirement savings plans are already exempt from taxes, a practice that Peterson and the Concord Coalition would like to encourage.
In effect, one form of income transfer to high earners (a tax subsidy
for private retirement savings) is being substituted for another (a
Social Security check).

For purposes here, however, the chief concern is that, with a
means test, Social Security would cross the boundary from entitlement
to charity. Once it is crossed, old-age assistance would become subject
to the same downward pressure as other means-tested programs, such
as AFDC (see Kingson and Quadagno, this volume). Support for
Social Security among middle- and upper-income groups would erode
with time, and in the long term, lower-income workers would suffer.

The Heart of the Matter: America's Bifurcated Welfare State

The additional distinctive feature of U.S. social provision lies in the
fact that while the United States embraced universality (social insurance and national standards) for elderly people, it left the working-age
population to rely mainly on programs of public charity and state-set
standards. Medicaid, Temporary Assistance for Needy Families (the
further devolved public assistance program that replaced AFDC in

1996), and unemployment insurance (an insurance program that is contractually based but administered according to state standards) have each been affected by fiscal competition among the states, which has eroded their value since the 1970s.

This bifurcation of welfare programs by age was by design. As Blank (1994) points out, Lyndon Johnson's *Economic Report of the President (1964)*, which laid out the intellectual foundations for his War on Poverty, emphasizes economic self-sufficiency. Improved schooling, housing, and job opportunities augmented by civil rights legislation would create what Quadagno (1994) calls the "equal opportunity welfare state." Employment, not transfers, would provide the solution to poverty. Government initiatives took the form of programs to improve the earnings opportunities for individuals—Head Start, education grants, job training, public health, community action programs—not more income transfers or public services. The exception was, of course, social provision for elderly people. The enactment of Medicare in 1965, liberalizations in OASI benefits, and later, indexing those benefits to inflation resulted in major new protections for old people, all in the form of social insurance transfers. Based on postwar experience, President Johnson's advisers had good reason for this strategy. From the 1940s through the 1960s, the U.S. economy brought dramatic gains in real living standards for the working-age population. Trends in wages and earnings in the 1940s and 1950s brought more, not less, equality (Goldin and Margo 1992). And, fueled by an expanding labor movement, more and more workers were gaining security (pensions, health care) through their employers.

In the 1980s, however, this employment-driven model failed. Despite a strong economic recovery after 1983, real wages and earnings unexpectedly declined among the bottom half of the labor market. Income inequality and child poverty rose sharply in the United States. Because the effects of wage polarization were experienced mainly by young adults, younger children were especially vulnerable. In Canada, where a more transfer-intensive model was adopted in the 1960s, this decline in aggregate social welfare did not appear, despite similar trends in labor market income (see Myles 1995 for a review of the literature).

The political consequences of these developments have been curious, to say the least. Market failure became interpreted as welfare state failure. Critics such as Charles Murray (1984) blamed rising child poverty on Johnson's Great Society programs, even though these programs were designed to enhance employment opportunities rather than to foster welfare dependency. Even more curious, at least to outsiders, was the emergence in the United States (and only in the United States) of the so-called generational equity debate. Because old-age poverty did not rise along with child poverty in the 1980s, Social Security and "greedy grannies" were spuriously held responsible for the new problems of the young. Oddly ignored throughout this time was the real rise in incomes and assets of middle-aged Americans in the top third of the income distribution.

A New Contract for Tomorrow's Old People?

Because of the failure of the market, since the 1970s, to deliver good jobs at decent wage, both charity (public assistance) and contract (old-age entitlements) are now under attack. The absence of a discourse of social citizenship and social rights means that those who would defend Social Security (or improve family benefits) have few rhetorical tools at their disposal. Rights cannot be violated, but contracts can be rewritten.

The great irony in all this is that those who will be affected by a revised Social Security contract are the young, not the old. The elderly people of today are not the concern. Their fate has been largely sealed by decisions taken in the past and by their own economic biographies. Although there may be modest tinkering around the margins of provisions relevant to today's elderly people, the main targets of any substantial Social Security reform taken today are the baby boomers and those following behind them. And these are the very people who have already borne the brunt of almost two decades of market failure and rising inequality. Generation X has every reason to be concerned, but we should be very precise in isolating the source of that concern, lest we make matters worse.

We can safely project that inequality among future generations of elderly people (those now in the labor force) will be greater than today. The divisions that have grown in the labor market since the 1970s will carry forward into the retirement years. Workers in part-time and low-wage employment are not accumulating the pension credits they require for retirement. This development will be exacerbated by the high divorce rate among this generation of adults. The breakdown of marriage typically brings a substantial reduction in income for women, one that they will carry forward to their retirement years.

The partial privatization of Old Age Insurance via a means test will exacerbate this development. If there is one thing we have learned from pension research in the past decade, it is that a private-public mix in retirement benefits has a major impact on the level of inequality in old age. The greater the share of old-age income that comes from private pensions and investments, the greater the inequality, since the distribution of market-based income is always larger than public sector benefits (Korpi and Palme 1994; Smeeding, Torrey, and Rainwater 1993).

Conclusion

Many observers of the 1950s and 1960s saw the more expansive understanding of democracy implicit in the extension of the welfare state as a natural and virtually irreversible feature of modernity and of the modern state. Social rights and the welfare state were simply the next logical step in a process of democratic reform that had been unfolding since the seventeenth century.

Marshall, however, was far less certain about all this. He noted that the emergence of social rights posed a curious paradox, since it coincided exactly with the rise of capitalism—a system not of equality but of inequality. As Marshall and others have pointed out from the beginning, social rights are different. Whereas civil rights are chiefly rights against the state, social rights are claims for protection by the state against markets and the rights of property. To guarantee social rights to all, we must impose limits on, perhaps even violate, property rights. The underdevelopment of the social rights tradition in U.S. political life lies at the heart of this conflict. This underdevelopment has not only precluded the development of citizen benefits in the United States but also has made possible the erosion of age-based citizen-worker benefits, which were substantially liberalized in the 1960s and 1970s.

Underlying the debates over universality, in all of its meanings, is a more fundamental debate about the nature and limits of democratic citizenship. To point out this fact does not resolve the debate but may help remind us of what the debate is about.

References

Blank, R. 1994. The Employment Strategy: Public Policies to Increase Work and Earnings. In S. Danziger, G. Sandefur, and D. Weinburg, eds., *Con-*

fronting Poverty: Prescriptions for Change. Cambridge: Harvard University Press.

Fraser, N., and L. Gordon. 1992. Contract versus Charity: Why Is There No Social Citizenship in the United States. *Socialist Review* 22:45–67.

Goldin, C., and R. Margo. 1992. The Great Compression: The Wage Structure of the United States at Mid-Century. *Quarterly Journal of Economics* 107:1–34.

Korpi, W., and J. Palme. 1994. *The Strategy of Equality and the Paradox of Redistribution.* Stockholm: Swedish Institute for Social Research.

Marshall, T. 1964. *Class, Citizenship, and Social Development.* Chicago: University of Chicago Press.

Murray, C. 1984. *Losing Ground: American Social Policy, 1950–1980.* New York: Basic Books.

Myles, J. 1995. *When Markets Fail: Social Welfare in Canada and the United States.* Geneva: United Nations Research Institute for Social Development.

Osberg, L. 1992. *The Economics of National Standards.* Halifax, Nova Scotia: Dalhousie University Press.

Peterson, P. 1993. *Facing Up: How to Rescue the Economy from Crushing Debt and Restore the American Dream.* New York: Simon and Schuster.

Peterson, P., and M. Rom. 1988. The Case for a National Welfare Standard. *Brookings Review* 6:24–32.

Quadagno, J. 1994. *The Color of Welfare: How Racism Undermined the War on Poverty.* New York: Oxford University Press.

Skocpol, T. 1992. *Protecting Soldiers and Mothers: The Origins of Social Policy in the United States.* Cambridge: Harvard University Press.

Smeeding, T., B. Torney, and L. Rainwater. 1993. Going to Extremes: An International Perspective on the U.S. Aged. Working Paper 87, Luxembourg Income Study.

Tiebout, C. 1956. A Pure Theory of Local Expenditures. *Journal of Political Economy* (Oct.): 416–24.

5

The Old-Age Lobby in a
New Political Era

ROBERT H. BINSTOCK

During the mid-1990s the political focus of old-age interest groups in the United States shifted from offense to defense. Throughout 1993 and much of 1994, these organizations were politically energized by the promise of a new multibillion-dollar federal program for home and community long-term care services that was part of President Bill Clinton's broad proposal for health care reform. The Clinton proposal failed, and the promise faded. Now these same interest groups are faced with the challenge of how to protect the thirty-year-old Medicare and Medicaid programs from substantial reductions in funding and from significant structural changes.

Initiatives undertaken by Congress that began in 1995 made it dramatically clear that there is a new era in the politics of aging. Proposed changes in federal policies on aging are now part of a sweeping agenda for limiting the role of government, redistributing the responsibilities of the federal government to state governments, and bringing the annual federal budget into balance. During earlier periods in the twentieth century, the political milieu of policies on aging was framed much more by the status of older people and the efficacy of programs designed to serve them.

This chapter explores the new political context of policies on aging and responses to it by the old-age lobby, those interest groups that seek to preserve the major role of the federal government in pro-

viding benefits to older persons. After a brief review of the politics of
aging in earlier eras, it examines the new era and the possible consequences of the changes in old-age programs that are contemplated by
Congress. Then it analyzes the strategic options that the interest
groups have for responding to the proposed changes, with particular
attention to the choices available to the thirty-three-million-member
American Association of Retired Persons (AARP). A brief concluding
section speculates about how needs within the older population might
come to be most effectively represented politically in the late 1990s
and beyond.

Policies and Interest Groups in the Earlier Eras

From the New Deal of the 1930s through the 1970s, older Americans
were compassionately stereotyped by the media as poor, frail, dependent, and above all, deserving (Binstock 1983). The American polity
responded to this compassionate construct by establishing the Social
Security program, Medicare, the Older Americans Act, the Employee
Retirement Income Security Act, special tax exemptions and credits
simply for being age sixty-five or older, and many additional measures.
Most programs that provided benefits and protection to older people
were structured primarily on the basis of old age, without much reference to variations in economic well-being, health status, and social
conditions within the older population, thereby creating what has
been termed an old-age welfare state (Myles 1983).

The major policy innovations in these decades, such as Social
Security and Medicare, were established largely through the initiatives
of elites: national political leaders, reformers, and professionals. The
impact of old-age interest groups in creating policy was confined to
programs that distributed benefits to professionals and practitioners in
the field of aging rather than directly to older people, themselves (see
Binstock and Day 1996). Indeed, the rise of many old-age political organizations mostly followed, rather than preceded and influenced, the
creation of government programs benefiting older people. Government
policies have provided both political and material incentives (including
hundreds of millions of dollars in direct grants and contracts) that
have fostered the formation and maintenance of old-age interest
groups (see Hudson 1995; Pratt 1993).

Starting in the late 1970s and continuing into the mid-1990s, new
stereotypes emerged in the popular culture depicting older people as

Differentiate
-Grants-in-aid
=Block-grants

prosperous, hedonistic, selfish, and politically powerful "greedy geezers." The most important factor contributing to this reversal of stereotypes was that academicians (e.g., Hudson 1978) and journalists (e.g., Samuelson 1978) began to recognize a tremendous growth trend in the proportion of government dollars expended on benefits to older Americans, which by 1995 exceeded one-third of the annual federal budget (U.S. Congress 1995). Comparisons between expenditures on older people and other social and economic causes began to emerge and were thematically unified and publicized as issues of so-called intergenerational equity by organizations such as Americans for Generational Equity (see Quadagno 1989) and the Concord Coalition (1993). The theme of intergenerational equity and conflict was adopted by the media, and by many academics and policy makers, as a routine perspective for describing many social policy issues (Cook et al. 1994).

Within this political climate of the 1980s and early 1990s, the age-categorical principle for distributing benefits and burdens among older people through programs on aging eroded substantially. Starting in 1983, Congress made a number of incremental changes in Social Security, Medicare, the Older Americans Act, and other programs and policies reflecting the diverse economic situations of older people (Binstock 1994). Some of these reduced benefits to comparatively wealthy older people; others targeted benefits toward relatively poor older people.

In this era, the activities of old-age interest groups were aimed at protecting existing programs and their specific features. These defensive efforts were somewhat successful in the broad sense that cutbacks in old-age programs during this period were generally less than in other social programs. Nonetheless, Congress did introduce a number of means tests and other measures that made policies on aging reflect more fully the diverse economic situations of older people.

The New Political Context for Policies on Aging

The new era of aging politics that emerged in the mid-1990s is distinct from the previous eras in two fundamental respects. First, it is shaped predominantly by a political agenda larger than one concerned only with the status of older people or even issues of intergenerational equity. Second, the reforms being proposed for programs affecting older Americans may have substantial and grave consequences for large segments of present and future elderly populations, especially those among them who are not well-off economically. This possibility is in stark contrast to the effects of the minor incremental policy changes enacted in the 1980s and early 1990s.

The larger political agenda introduced by the 104th Congress is structured by the following basic principles that have long been staples of conservative ideology. First, government should play a less intrusive role than it now does in American society and in the lives of individuals. Second, citizens and businesses can make more effective use of their money if it remains in their hands, as opposed to being taken away through taxation to support governmental activities. And third, intricate social programs funded by federal grants-in-aid should be administered with substantial discretionary authority by state governments. As the 1996 election drew near, President Clinton expressed his general agreement with these principles by frequently proclaiming "the end of big government as we know it" and signing legislation (the Personal Responsibility and Work Opportunity Reconciliation Act of 1996) that effectively transferred the federal Aid to Families with Dependent Children welfare program to the states.

In addition, Republicans and many Democrats are acting on the principle that the annual budget of the federal government should be brought into balance by sharply reducing expenditures. This concern for balancing the budget has already weighed heavily in proposals to make large reductions in projected Medicare and Medicaid expenditures and to make significant structural changes in the programs.

Medicare

Medicare outlays are projected to increase from $196 billion in fiscal year 1996 to $329 billion in 2002 (U.S. Congress 1996a). Moreover, the issue of how to pay for Medicare is rather immediate. Annual expenditures for Medicare's Part A Hospital Insurance (HI) already exceed substantially the revenues from the payroll tax that finances it, and HI trust fund reserves are being drawn upon to bridge the gap. A mid-1996 report of the Trustees of the Social Security Trust Fund estimates that the fund's reserves will be exhausted early in 2001 (Rosenbaum 1996).

In 1995 Congress submitted to President Clinton a budget bill for fiscal year 1996 that included a $270 billion reduction in projected Medicare spending by 2002. Although the president was willing to approve a smaller Medicare reduction, he vetoed the bill, citing the size of the reduction and the structural changes proposed for the program as among his reasons for doing so. In 1996 Congress developed a budget resolution for reductions of $153 billion in projected Medicare spending between 1997 and 2002 (U.S. Congress 1996b); President Clinton proposed $72 billion in reductions over the same period (Wines 1996). When the election season drew near, however, no legislative action was taken. Yet the strategies that the 104th Congress envisioned for achieving reductions are likely to shape the agenda for Medicare reform for the rest of the decade.

The general approach that appears to be favored is a transition from Medicare's traditional, open-ended, fee-for-service approach to a situation in which most of Medicare operates within fixed budgets that cap program costs. The various strategies envisioned for carrying out this approach pose possible adverse consequences for segments of the older population. One strategy is to encourage the proliferation of—and enrollment in—Medicare managed care plans, such as health maintenance organizations (HMOs), which receive a flat per capita fee for providing health care for each beneficiary enrolled in the plan. The financial incentives of managed care organizations, however, foster the undertreatment of patients (see Kane and Kane 1994). Nothing in the experience of more than a decade of Medicare HMO experiments launched by the federal Health Care Financing Administration is reassuring on this score, because enrollees in these programs have tended to be relatively healthy older persons (see Brown et al. 1993), and even they seem to have been underserved in certain respects (Wiener and Skaggs 1995).

A second strategy is to establish individual tax-exempt medical savings accounts (MSAs): under this plan, each Medicare participant would receive from Medicare an annual flat sum, part of it to purchase a high-deductible catastrophic health insurance policy and part of it to purchase health care. Unused balances in such accounts would be retained by Medicare participants, to be spent or invested or even passed on through inheritance. Most policy analysts expect that relatively healthy and wealthy older people would opt for MSAs. But it is also a distinct possibility that poorer older people would also select the MSA option. The sum paid into their MSAs by Medicare may be perceived as a cash windfall by those older people either below the poverty line or only a few thousand dollars above it. These poor old people may well forgo needed medical care in order to preserve the windfall, even though poor old people tend to be relatively unhealthy (Robert and House 1994); a consequence could be that they would need even more health care if and when they finally do seek it.

A third strategy is to set a projected annual spending cap for aggregate reimbursements for the traditional fee-for-service portion of Medicare. If spending exceeds the cap, a fail-safe mechanism would enforce the target by reducing reimbursement rates to health care providers in order to make up for the aggregate excess spending. This, in turn, would likely have an impact on the quality of care received by Medicare patients—as well as by other patients. For instance, cutbacks in hospital reimbursements would lead to deterioration in the facilities, equipment, and staff services available for patients of all ages.

Medicaid

Between 1989 and 1995 Medicaid expenditures for long-term care grew at an annualized rate of 13.2 percent (U.S. General Accounting Office 1995). In 1995 Congress initially proposed to cap the rate of growth in Medicaid expenditures in order to achieve savings of $182 billion by 2002, to eliminate federal requirements for determining individual eligibility for Medicaid (as an entitlement), and to turn over control of the program to state governments through capped block grants. President Clinton's veto of the budget bill killed this proposal, but it resurfaced in 1996 with proposed reductions totaling $72 billion (U.S. Congress 1996b).

This approach for changing Medicaid remains on the policy agenda, strongly supported by the bipartisan National Governors Conference. If it becomes law, state governments would have to face a number of critical allocative issues. The resolution of these issues would vary, of course, from state to state, but it seems likely that, throughout the states, Medicaid spending on long-term care would be much less than is projected at present. Under present law Medicaid pays for the care, at least in part, of about three-fifths of nursing home patients (Wiener and Illston 1996) and 28 percent of home and community services (AARP 1994).

One decision that states will have to face is whether to make up from their own funds the difference between the federal funds they would have received under current law and the lower amounts (after the first year of the new program) that they will receive in the form of block grants. According to one analysis (Kassner 1995), the 1995 congressional proposal for a Medicaid block grant would have trimmed long-term care funding by as much as 11.4 percent by 2000, which means that 1.74 million Medicaid beneficiaries would have lost—or have been unable to secure—coverage. It is unlikely that any states will provide their own funds to compensate for such a gap in federal funding. State expenditures on Medicaid are already 20 percent of the budget in some states and are growing fast in almost all states.

A second decision is whether to maintain the present level of expenditure, and perhaps keep up with health care cost inflation, for the state's own share of Medicaid funding. This would be politically and budgetarily difficult in many states. Most state constitutions require that the state budget (unlike the federal budget) must be balanced. It is possible, of course, that Congress will follow the precedent it set in 1996, when it transformed AFDC into a block grant program but required the states to maintain at least 75–80 percent of their current Medicaid funding in order to receive federal grants.

The decisions of most states on these two issues—making up the federal funding gap and maintaining present state levels of funding—are likely to result in shrinking Medicaid resources for long-term care. Medicaid funding of home and community care may disappear in some states and be cut back severely in others. Rates of reimbursement to nursing homes may, at best, be held constant, which would have the effect of ratcheting them down because of ongoing inflation in the costs of providing nursing home care.

A third issue that the states will confront is how to allocate limited and shrinking resources among the categorical groups eligible for Medicaid—the aged, the disabled, and single mothers and children. This issue, unfortunately, is likely to engender heated political conflict among advocates of the respective constituents in these groups.

In tandem with this is a fourth set of decisions. States would have to set income and asset eligibility standards for Medicaid applications, to replace the minimum federal entitlement standards that may be eliminated under a block grant program. Some states that now employ the minimum required levels may well set their criteria at lower levels, drastically reducing the number of persons eligible for Medicaid. Those that currently have more generous levels than the federal minimum may also be tempted to reduce the pool of Medicaid participants when faced with a cap on federal grant funds.

Underlying these four issues that states would confront is a very fundamental policy question: How does the state intend to deal with functionally disabled elders and younger people who have no place to turn—persons who cannot afford to pay for long-term care out of pocket, are not eligible for Medicaid, and do not have access to informal care from family and friends? This has always been an implicit issue, of course, but in the context of Medicaid block grants, it would need to become explicit and urgent, especially in those states that (1) do not choose to make up for the gap in federal funding, (2) do not maintain state funding levels at an adequate rate, (3) curtail the portion of Medicaid funds available to elderly persons (as opposed to other categories of Medicaid eligibility), and (4) tighten the income and asset eligibility standards.

In sum, it seems likely that turning Medicaid into a block grant would substantially weaken the long-term care safety net that Medicaid provides for older people and their families (as well as other constituencies). Some analysts predict that substantial reductions in current state Medicaid spending will almost certainly occur unless federal law requires states to increase their funding for the program (e.g., U.S. General Accounting Office 1995a, 1995b) and that nascent home and community services would be decimated in at least half of the states (e.g., Kassner 1995).

Old-Age Interest Groups in the New Political Context

As manifested in these Medicare and Medicaid proposals, the new era in the politics of policies on aging poses difficult challenges for old-age interest groups that purport to be vigorous and effective advocates for a strong federal role in promoting the well-being of older people. These groups (the old-age lobby) registered concerns about the propositions for reducing and reorganizing Medicare and Medicaid as early as 1994 (Toner 1994). But what will be their responses in the late 1990s to proposals for these and other significant cutbacks and changes in programs on aging? How much emphasis will they give to the plight of the poor elderly as opposed to concerns for all older Americans? Will they attempt to ally with and represent younger constituencies that would be adversely affected by program changes? Will they invest far greater resources in lobbying efforts than they have in the past, and undertake confrontational tactics, in an all-out effort to succeed? Will they be willing to employ political strategies that may have a probability of immediate success but that may jeopardize their long-run organizational viability? Or will they merely attempt to establish a clear record that they are fighting the good fight, win or lose? Actions taken and not taken during 1995 and 1996, as well as analyses of these interest groups, provide a basis for addressing these questions.

The most important responses to the old-age policy challenges of the mid-1990s and beyond will be those undertaken by mass-membership old-age organizations that seek to preserve the old-age welfare state, particularly the AARP. (Those organizations that seek to reduce the role of the federal government are discussed later in this chapter.) To be sure, there are dozens of interest groups focused on issues of aging (see Day 1995; Van Tassel and Meyer 1992), forty-one of which constitute the Leadership Council of Aging Organizations. For those that are not based on mass memberships, however, the choices of political strategy will be relatively straightforward, and their impact is likely to be small in the present political context.

Single-issue groups such as those focused on older women (e.g., the Older Women's League) and various ethnic and racial subgroups of older people (e.g., the National Caucus and Center on the Black Aged) will undoubtedly identify specific ways in which proposed program changes will adversely affect their respective constituencies. These groups are likely to lobby Congress armed with policy analyses highlighting their concerns for their subgroups, which are predominantly poor (this was their approach during the 104th Congress). Whether or not these groups form a coalition, their effectiveness tends to be very limited because they have neither the capacity to mobilize mass constituencies nor broad support from state and local politicians.

Professional organizations concerned with aging-related research and education are similarly hamstrung by their lack of resources for exercising political influence, and they are not, in any event, focused primarily on the plight of relatively poor older people. With respect to the proposed changes in Medicare and Medicaid, they will have no strategic choices to make other than to decide whether to express solidarity with other interest groups in the old-age lobby. They will, of course, take the lead in attempting to fend off proposals to eliminate or cut back programs for research and education, as they did in 1995 regarding legislation that affected the National Institute on Aging, Title IV of the Older Americans Act, and the Agency for Health Care Policy Research.

Trade organizations that serve older people as clients and customers will focus on the likely impacts upon their respective industries rather than on the effects on older people per se. These organizations will draw upon their state and local political connections, as well as the older people whom they serve, to protest possible cutbacks and other adverse changes in the programs that sustain their operations. This strategy has had some success over the years. In early 1995, for instance, such protests led Congress to scrap its plan to enfold funds that are currently earmarked for congregate and home-delivered meals for the elderly into a broad nutrition block grant to the states (see "Senior Power Rides Again," *Newsweek*, February 20, 1995).

The Special Case of the AARP

The most difficult and politically important choices will be those made by the AARP. Although it is only one of some half-dozen old-age mass-membership organizations (see Van Tassel and Meyer 1992), it is by far the most important because of its huge membership (more than three times larger than the combined total of all the others), its vastly superior financial and staff resources, and its reputation in Washington as the most politically powerful of the age-based groups. In addition to the implicit political clout of having thirty-three million members of voting age, the AARP has substantial financial resources to undergird its political activities. In 1994, its total revenues were $469 million, consisting of $146 million from membership dues, $102 million from group health insurance, $86 million in federal grants and contracts, $47 million from advertising in its publications, $24 million in interest income, and $64 million from other activities such as a prescription drug service, mutual funds, credit cards, travel services, and auto, homeowner's, and life insurance (Pear 1995). The organization has 1,700 employees and about 250,000 trained volunteers ("GOP Senator Investigates Finances of Retirees' Group," *New York Times*, April 9, 1995). It maintains about four thousand local chapters, which are more social than political in nature and include about 3 percent of the membership (Day 1995). It operates a public policy research institute. And it engages heavily in political lobbying.

Whatever AARP chooses to do (or not do) tends to define the overall position of the old-age lobby. By the same token, the strategies of the rest of the organizations (including mass- membership organizations) tend to be politically insignificant if the AARP does not take the lead on them.

As the AARP develops its lobbying strategy, it is constrained by an overriding consideration, namely, that its political views and strategies should not alienate substantial portions of the membership, which pays dues and buys products and services marketed by the organization. The organization's staff and volunteer leaders have long recognized that the membership is diverse in political views, and they try to avoid taking stands on what they regard as "hopelessly divisive issues, for example, euthanasia" (Rother 1995a).

There have been two occasions in recent years, however, when the AARP's political stances have noticeably antagonized some segments of its membership. In 1988 the AARP endorsed the Medicare Catastrophic Coverage Act, which levied a sliding-scale income surtax on relatively well-off older people to pay for new hospital insurance benefits. A great many members of the organization registered strong protests to the tax through public demonstrations and through telephone calls and written communications to congressional representatives. In response, Congress quickly repealed the surtax, despite the AARP's ongoing support for the legislation (see Binstock and Murray 1991; Crystal 1990; Day 1993). Substantial dissent was also registered in 1994 when the AARP announced support for the Democratic leadership's health care reform bills in the Senate and the House (see "Endorsement Riles Members of Retiree Group," *New York Times*, August 12, 1994; "Not All in AARP Are behind Health Care Plan," *New York Times*, August 13, 1994). On both occasions it was rumored that a small minority of members had resigned. These episodes were not major blows to the organization. Nonetheless, following the defeat of health care reform in the 103d Congress, the president of the AARP publicly acknowledged that his membership had widely divergent and strongly held views and that representing a diverse membership in public policy affairs is an ongoing struggle for the organization (Lehrman 1995).

Because the changes proposed in Medicare and Medicaid are likely to have the greatest adverse effects on the poorest and the near-poor elderly, the AARP is faced with an important choice regarding how much priority it should give to concerns for low-income older people in the substance of its advocacy positions. It could, for example, suggest to Congress policy alternatives that embody measures for minimizing harm to poor elders, while trading off other aspects of the two programs. Yet, a strategy of this kind would be likely to anger a sizable portion of middle- and upper-income members of the organization. Over the years, the AARP has given attention to the needs of low-income older people through legislative testimony, letters to Congress, outreach programs, policy analyses, and various other advocacy efforts. But if the organization chooses to give primary attention to the plight of the poor in the context of major changes in Medicare and Medicaid, it will not be representing its membership so much as championing a more circumscribed social cause.

An alternative path, of course, would be to defend the status quo more generally, although this strategy needs to include a recognition that some short-term changes in Medicare's Part A Hospital Insurance program are needed if it is to meet its expenditure obligations in 2001. AARP's director of legislation and public policy has acknowledged that, because of the imminent shortfall in Part A, his organization will probably have to give some ground in defending Medicare in order to maintain its credibility in policy debates (Anderson and Binstein 1995). In this context, the AARP can still point out that Medicare's universal coverage serves poor older people very well (much as Social Security does), an advocacy stance for which the AARP laid the groundwork in 1995 (Carlson 1995). Medicaid can be depicted as an essential safety net not only for the poor but also for deserving middle-class older people who have "spent down" their assets on long-term care. These stances would probably represent the views of most members and would thereby be safe in terms of organizational maintenance. They were expressed in 1995 with no apparent backlash from the membership.

The AARP also has to decide whether to include in its focus the interests of other constituencies, which are not elderly, with which it might form coalitions. For example, if it chooses to emphasize the concerns of low-income elders, natural allies with respect to Medicaid issues would be organizations representing the poor, the disabled, and ethnic and racial minorities of all ages. Again, this approach might generate considerable disaffection within AARP's membership. No major coalitional efforts of this kind were undertaken in 1995 and 1996.

Still another choice confronting the AARP is whether it should engage in its customary lobbying tactics or whether the organization's reputational and financial resources should be very heavily invested in either conventional or relatively militant political activities. AARP's traditional approach has shown little capacity to cohere the votes or other political activities of older people (see Binstock and Day 1996), despite the organization's huge membership, its reputation for political power, and its well-financed lobbying apparatus.

As implied above, in the 1980s and early 1990s the AARP was ineffective in attempting to fend off various changes in policies on aging, such as the elimination in 1986 of the extra personal exemption from federal income taxes that was available to all people age sixty-five and older and the repeal of the Medicare Catastrophic Coverage Act in 1989. In the early 1980s the AARP opposed the proposition that Social Security benefits be taxed for middle- and high-income retirees but capitulated in 1983, when a presidential commission recommended it as part of a package of Social Security reforms. In 1993, when additional taxation of Social Security benefits was enacted, little was heard from the AARP. The 1995 congressional budget resolution could have been used by the AARP to construct "tabloid symbols" (Allport 1959) that would have been rallying points for more effective lobbying: "Medicare and Medicaid cuts total $452 billion!" "Block grants to states for Medicaid cause low-quality care in nursing homes and the demolition of home care programs!" Such a strategy, along with massive investments of staff and money, could have been used to launch a major media campaign, produce tens of millions of letters to members of the Senate and House, organize political action committees, hold rallies in congressional districts, and undertake other relatively conventional lobbying tactics far more robustly than the AARP has in the past. An additional, unconventional tactic would have been to organize mammoth, militant, sit-in protests with tens of thousands of elderly persons (and perhaps other constituencies).

But the AARP did not take this approach. In the summer of 1995, it did announce a "nationwide, grassroots campaign" to celebrate the thirtieth anniversary of Medicare, consisting of "30 events in 30 states" (AARP 1995). These events drew crowds ranging from one hundred to five hundred persons, were not particularly militant, and except for the kickoff event at the Lyndon Baines Johnson Library in Texas, received no attention from the national media.

The primary approach taken by the AARP in response to the 1995 budget bill was relatively modest and inconspicuous. Its staff and lay leaders met periodically with members of Congress and congressional staff in attempts to reverse selected elements in the budget bill. For example, they tried to stop a proposed elimination of federal regulation of quality of care in nursing homes (Rother 1995b). Yet, even on this matter, the language in the final bill did not preclude such regulation from being effectively eliminated.

Overall, one suspects that the AARP will be relatively conservative in its choices. It will probably choose to defend the status quo as best it can rather than give top priority to concerns for elderly poor people. It is unlikely to form alliances with non-age-based interests representing poor people, disabled people, and ethnic and racial minorities. Its tactical approach will probably be relatively moderate, forgoing massive investments in conventional lobbying approaches and eschewing efforts at militant activities that would involve mobilizing large numbers of older people to express protests through their immediate physical presence.

The major reason that the AARP is likely to make conservative choices is that it has been and will continue to be guided by the fundamental imperative of organizational survival. From the perspective of the classic literature on political organizations (Clark and Wilson 1961; Wilson 1973), the AARP is an organization that maintains itself primarily through the material and associational incentives it provides to its members, rather than through political incentives. Day (1995, 8) concludes from her research that "AARP is the quintessential example" of such an organization. Indeed, in 1996 the AARP launched a major initiative to license managed care health plans in order to maintain its substantial role in the health insurance business (see Freudenheim 1996). Seen in this light, the political activities of the organization can be interpreted as membership marketing strategies. In short, the incentive system of the organization dictates that it defend old-age programs against major changes but that this fight, win or lose, does not include positions and tactics that jeopardize the organization's membership and financial resources.

Another reason that the AARP is likely to be restrained in its choices is that it has come under attack by several U.S. senators who have proposed major benefit reductions in Social Security and anticipate opposition from AARP. Two Senate hearings were held in 1995 at which various witnesses criticized AARP's organizational practices and its tax-exempt status (e.g., Goldberg 1995; Hewitt 1995; Olson 1995). Senator Simpson of Wyoming charged that the AARP had "drifted considerably from any reasonable description of a nonprofit organization that should enjoy a tax exemption and unlimited lobbying privileges"; he also asserted that the organization "imposes a policy agenda on an unwilling membership" (Pear 1995). These hearings, and the media coverage of them, somewhat tarnished the legitimacy of the AARP as an advocate for older people, generated uncertainty regarding its ongoing tax-exempt status, raised questions about the propriety of its lobbying of the federal government when in one year alone it received $86 million in federal grants, and opened up a wider discussion of lobbying by tax-exempt organizations, in general (e.g., "Why Stop with the AARP?" *New York Times*, June 16, 1995). Further attacks, including proposed legislation to revise tax exemptions, remain a distinct threat, especially if the Republicans maintain control of Congress.

Conclusion

A new era in the politics of aging, which began to take shape in the early 1990s (Hudson 1993), had emerged in full bloom by the middle of the decade. Proposals for major changes in programs on aging are being generated by conservative political principles and by efforts to balance the federal budget, without much attention to the implications for older people themselves. In addition to proposals for substantially restructuring and reducing projected expenditures in the Medicare and Medicaid programs, major proposals for reforming Social Security—including efforts to privatize that program—are almost certain to emerge on the legislative agenda in the late 1990s (see Dreyfuss 1996; Quadagno 1996).

In responding to these kinds of policy change, the old-age interest groups that advocate a strong role for the federal government in programs on aging will have some important choices to make regarding the substance of their positions, the formation of strategic alliances, and political tactics. The key decisions will be those made by the AARP, because it has far greater potential for exercising political influence than do the others. The more radical options might have some effects on the outcome of legislative deliberations, but the AARP will probably opt for the more traditional choices, impelled by its internal incentive system and, perhaps, influenced by congressional inquiries regarding its tax-exempt status.

Consequently, the old-age lobby is unlikely to have much impact unless its efforts are coincidentally fortified by more powerful political forces. Traditionally, the consumer orientation of many old-age organizations has often put them at odds with health care providers. Yet, with respect to proposals for changes in Medicare and Medicaid, hospitals, nursing homes, physicians, and other health care providers have major financial stakes in preserving as much of the status quo as they can (see Clymer 1995; Toner 1995a). Hence, the old-age and health care interests may become strange bedfellows in this new era in the politics of aging and thus have some combined effect on the details of reforms.

At the same time, however, the Republican Medicare and Medicaid proposals are being supported by a broad range of business interests, which have formed a Coalition to Save Medicare. This coalition includes the United States Chamber of Commerce, the National Association of Manufacturers, the National Restaurant Association, the Alliance for Managed Care (representing large insurance companies), the National Taxpayers Union, and a recently established conservative front organization named the Seniors Coalition (Toner 1995b). The Seniors Coalition launched a direct-mail attack on the AARP, in which it proclaims, "We reject the tried-and-failed AARP policies of big government, deficit spending, and social engineering" (Seniors Coalition 1995). Through this strategy the Senior Coalition has joined three other organizations at the conservative end of the ideological spectrum—United Seniors Coalition, 60/Plus Association, and the National Alliance of Senior Citizens—that espouse "limited government in the area of social welfare, free market reforms, and partial or full privatization of old-age benefits" (Day 1995, 4).

Clearly, in the late 1990s the scope of political conflict affecting policies on aging is now much broader than it was in earlier eras. In this new era, the viability of old-age interest groups in effectively representing a heterogeneous population of older people may become increasingly problematic. Not only are older people going to remain diverse with respect to social and economic characteristics and political leanings, but age differences within the older population may become more important politically. In the years ahead the AARP (which solicits membership among people age fifty and older) and other mass-membership old-age organizations will have baby boomers joining their ranks. The old-age lobby may find that its younger members tend to support substantial contemporary changes in Medicare, Medicaid, and Social Security to preserve the long-run viability of these programs, while older cohorts may wish to preserve present program features and have relatively little concern for longer-run consequences.

As the twentieth century comes to a close, the older population may come to be most effectively represented by a new and broad constellation of interest groups that is ideologically committed to promoting the role of the federal government in fostering the well-being of people of all ages within American society. Perhaps the AARP and other old-age interest groups will be part of such a coalition. If they are not, they may have little influence on major changes in social policies on aging.

References

AARP (American Association of Retired Persons). 1994. *The Costs of Long-Term Care.* Washington, D.C.
———. 1995. "AARP Announces Nationwide Campaign to Celebrate Thirty Years of Medicare." News release, July 27.
Allport, G. 1959. ABCs of Scapegoating. New York: Anti-Defamation League of B'nai B'rith.
Anderson, J., and M. Binstein. 1995. AARP's Medicare Debate Quandary. *Washington Post,* July 6.
Binstock, R. 1983. The Aged as Scapegoat. *Gerontologist* 23:136–43.
———. 1994. Changing Criteria in Old-Age Programs: The Introduction of Economic Status and Need for Services. *Gerontologist* 34:726–30.
Binstock, R., and C. Day. 1996. Aging and Politics. In R. Binstock and L. George, eds., *Handbook of Aging and the Social Sciences,* 4th ed. San Diego: Academic.
Binstock, R., and T. Murray. 1991. The Politics of Developing Appropriate Care for Dementia. In R. Binstock, S. Post, and P. Whitehouse, eds., *Dementia and Aging: Ethics, Values, and Policy Choices.* Baltimore: Johns Hopkins University Press.
Brown, R., J. Bergeron, D. Clement, J. Hill, and S. Rettchin. 1993. *Does Managed Care Work for Medicare? An Evaluation of the Medicare Risk Program for HMOs.* Princeton, N.J.: Mathematica Policy Research.
Carlson, E. 1995. Council Vows to Back Key Programs. *AARP Bulletin* 36(3): 1, 7–9.
Clark, P., and J. Wilson. 1961. Incentive Systems: A Theory of Organizations. *Administrative Science Quarterly* 6:219–66.
Clymer, A. 1995. Nursing Home Industry Looks Askance at Republican Plans to Cut Medicaid. *New York Times,* June 14.
Concord Coalition. 1993. *The Zero Deficit Plan: A Plan for Eliminating the Federal Budget Deficit by the Year 2000.* Washington, D.C.
Cook, F., D. Marshall, J. Marshall, and J. Kaufman. 1994. The Salience of Intergenerational Equity in Canada and the United States. In T. Marmor, T. Smeeding, and V. Greene, eds., *Economic Security and Intergenerational Justice: A Look at North America.* Washington, D.C.: Urban Institute.
Crystal, S. 1990. Health Economics, Old-Age Politics, and the Catastrophic Medicare Debate. *Journal of Gerontological Social Work* 15:21–31.
Day, C. 1993. Older Americans' Attitudes toward the Medicare Catastrophic Coverage Act of 1988. *Journal of Politics* 55:167–77.
———. 1995. Old-Age Interest Groups in the 1990s: Coalition, Competition, and Strategy. Paper presented at the annual meeting of the American Political Science Association, Chicago, Sept. 2.

Dreyfuss, R. 1996. The Biggest Deal: Lobbying to Make Social Security Private. *American Prospect* (May–June): 72–75.

Freudenheim, M. 1996. AARP Will License Its Name to Managed Health Care Plans. *New York Times*, Apr. 4.

Goldberg, M. 1995. Statement before the U.S. Senate Finance Committee, Subcommittee on Social Security and Family Policy, June 13.

Hewitt, P. 1995. Statement before the U.S. Senate Finance Committee, Subcommittee on Social Security and Family Policy, June 13.

Hudson, R. 1978. The "Graying" of the Federal Budget and Its Consequences for Old Age Policy. Gerontologist 18:428–40.

———. 1993. The "Graying" of the Federal Budget Revisited. *Generations* 17:79–82.

———. 1995. Old-Age Interest Groups in Comparative Perspective. *Gerontologist* 35:420–21.

Kane, R., and R. Kane. 1994. Effects of the Clinton Health Reform on Older Persons and Their Families: A Health Care Systems Perspective. *Gerontologist* 34:598–605.

Kassner, E. 1995. *Long-Term Care: Measuring the Impact of a Medicaid Cap.* Washington, D.C.: American Association of Retired Persons.

Lehrman, E. 1995. Health Care Reform at the Crossroads. *Modern Maturity* (Jan.–Feb.): 12.

Myles, J. 1983. Conflict, Crisis, and the Future of Old Age Security. *Milbank Memorial Fund Quarterly/Health and Society* 61:462–72.

Olson, M. 1995. Statement before the U.S. Senate Finance Committee, Subcommittee on Social Security and Family Policy, June 13.

Pear, R. 1995. Senator Challenges the Practices of a Retirees Association. *New York Times*, June 14.

Pratt, H. 1993. *Gray Agendas: Interest Groups and Public Pensions in Canada, Britain, and the United States.* Ann Arbor: University of Michigan Press.

Quadagno, J. 1989. Generational Equity and the Politics of the Welfare State. *Politics and Society* 17:353–76.

———. 1996. Social Security and the Myth of the Entitlement "Crisis." Gerontologist 36:391–99.

Robert, S., and J. House. 1994. Socioeconomic Status and Health over the Life Course. In R. Abeles, H. Gift, and M. Ory, eds., *Aging and the Quality of Life.* New York: Springer.

Rosenbaum, D. 1996. Gloomy Forecast Touches off Feud on Medicare Fund. *New York Times*, June 6.

Rother, J. 1995a. Written communication to author, Feb. 7.

———. 1995b. Medicare, Medicaid, and the Politics of Aging. Paper presented at the annual meeting of the Gerontological Society of America, Los Angeles, Nov. 17.

Samuelson, R. 1978. Aging America: Who Will Shoulder the Growing Burden? *National Journal* 10:1712–17.

Seniors Coalition. 1995. Undated direct-mail circular, circa July–Aug.

Toner, R. 1994. Groups Rally to Fight Medicare Cuts. *New York Times*, Dec. 18.

————. 1995a. Warning against Quick Medicare Cuts: Hospital Association Says the Republicans Are Moving Too Fast. *New York Times,* July 11.

————. 1995b. Medicare Battle Will Shift to Home Front. *New York Times,* Aug. 4.

U.S. Congress. 1995. *The Economic and Budget Outlook: Fiscal Years 1996–2000.* Washington, D.C.: Government Printing Office.

————. 1996a. *Reducing the Deficit: Spending and Revenue Options.* Washington, D.C.: Government Printing Office.

————. 1996b. *The Economic and Budget Outlook: An Update.* Washington, D.C.: Government Printing Office.

U.S. General Accounting Office. 1995. *Long-Term Care: Current Issues and Future Directions.* Washington, D.C.: Government Printing Office.

————. 1995. *Medicaid: Restructuring Approaches Leave Many Questions.* Washington, D.C.: Government Printing Office.

Van Tassel, D., and J. Meyer. 1992. *U.S. Aging Policy Interest Groups: Institutional Profiles.* New York: Greenwood.

Wiener, J., and L. Illston. 1996. Health Care Financing and Organization for the Elderly. In R. Binstock and L. George, eds., *Handbook of Aging and the Social Sciences,* 4th ed. San Diego: Academic.

Wiener, J., and S. Skaggs. 1995. *Current Approaches to Integrating Acute and Long-Term Care Financing and Services.* Washington, D.C.: American Association of Retired Persons.

Wilson, J. 1973. *Political Organizations.* New York: Basic Books.

Wines, M. 1996. Political Stakes Increase in Fight to Save Medicare. *New York Times,* June 3.

PART II

PUBLIC POLICY
AND POPULATION
DYNAMICS

6

The Emergence of the Oldest Old
Challenges for Public Policy

JUDITH G. GONYEA

The life course is a journey marked by stages. These life stages are not fixed; rather, they have over time expanded and shrunk in length, and new ones have emerged in response to broader social changes. This phenomenon is especially evident in the definition of *old age*. Before the late 1970s, all older Americans (typically defined as age sixty-five or older) were lumped together in a homogeneous grouping. It was not until the "democratization of aging"—that is, the new reality of the vast majority of Americans attaining old age and even advanced old age—that gerontologists began to differentiate between the young old, the old old, and the oldest old (Neugarten 1974; Harris 1978; Treas and Bengtson 1982).

Thus, the study of the oldest old is relatively new. It was only a short time ago that Suzman and Riley (1985, 177), as editors of a special issue of the *Milbank Quarterly* devoted to the topic of the oldest old, wrote that "less is known about it than any other age category" and that it is "so new a phenomenon that there is little in historical experience that can help in interpreting it." Yet, they also went on to predict that, given their rising numbers, the oldest old would "no longer remain invisible" in the economy, the polity, and the health and social service systems (ibid.). Indeed, the oldest old—variously defined as those over age seventy-five, eighty, and eighty-five—are now the fastest-growing segment of not only the aged population but also the overall U.S. population. In 1990, in the United States 6.9 million persons (or one in every thirty-five Americans) were age eighty or older. Those age one hundred or older doubled during the 1980s and numbered 35,808 Americans by 1990. Nor is this trend likely to change as the baby boomers—a cohort of 76 million persons born between 1946 and 1964—join the ranks of the elderly in the first half of the twenty-first century. The U.S. Bureau of the Census's (1992a) middle-series population projections (which assume 2.1 births per woman, an average life expectancy of 82.1 years by 2050, and net immigration of 800,000 by the turn of the century) estimate that the population age eighty and over will grow to more than 25 million persons (or one in every twelve Americans) by the year 2050. Moreover, it is projected that in 2050 centenarians will number 1,170,000.

The significance of the aging of the older population—and a yet faster-growing very old population—has not been lost on the world of public policy. Moreover, the public policy outlook has become increasingly dire, as referents have moved from "the graying of the federal budget" (Hudson 1978) to "a fiscal black hole" (Callahan 1987) to nothing less than "apocalyptic demographic forecasts" (Robertson 1991). Concomitantly, the long-held view of older people as "deserving" has come into question. In a typical example of the media view, *New York Times* columnist William Safire (May 15, 1995) wrote of borrowing to fund the growing deficit as "no longer . . . a gift to our old but a theft from our young."

The concerns about the extent of public spending on older people reflected in these comments are legitimate, if perhaps overstated. Nonetheless, they do ignore the significant gains in population well-being that have directly resulted from federal expenditures. Social Security has been central to the threefold drop, over a thirty-year period, in poverty among the aged; Medicare has brought acute health care coverage to virtually the entire older population, literally twice what it was in 1965; and Medicaid has funded vast amounts of intensive long-term care services. These comments ignore, as well, the particular areas of vulnerability associated with the recent and continuing rise of the oldest old.

As the following discussion makes clear, the oldest old are diverse. While they are least likely to fit the stereotype described by Binstock (1994)—"prosperous, hedonistic, selfish, and politically powerful," "greedy geezers"—neither are they inevitably poor, frail, and isolated. Still, there are considerable policy-related needs associated with very advanced age. The policy test lies in identifying individuals who have disabilities associated with very advanced age and asking (1) how policy responses can be better directed toward these needs and (2) whether such responses should be based on advanced chronological age alone or on functional status and income measures, which may apply to populations of all ages.

Diversity among the Oldest Old

Diversity among the oldest old has several dimensions.

Gender

It is immediately striking that the oldest old are predominately women. There are only forty-three males to every one hundred females age eighty-five to eighty-nine, and this gap widens by age one hundred to thirty males to every hundred females. Although it is often assumed that the aging (sixty and over) population has always been composed of mostly women, in fact until the 1930s males and females were almost equally represented among this age group. Both sexes benefited from improvements in nutrition, work and living environments, and medical therapies during the following sixty years, but gender-related morbidity and mortality risks paced the deaths differently. Whereas the proportion of older men rose from 4% to 10% of the population, the proportion of older women increased at a faster rate and now approaches 15% (Thompson 1994). Evidence suggests that by the year 2050, the gender gap in longevity may have peaked and will eventually level off to about forty-two men for every hundred women in the eighty-five and over age group (U.S. Bureau of the Census 1992a).

Income

Although in comparison to older women, older men experience a mortality disadvantage, they do have a quality-of-life advantage—particularly older white men (Longino 1988; Barer 1994). As Thompson (1994, 10) suggests, "death may come sooner, but later life for older men presents fewer problems." Table 6.1 presents the percentages of the poor and near poor by age, sex, and race or ethnicity for the older population in 1990. The interactive effects of gender, race, and age on the experience of poverty are reflected in the fact that the poorest group of elderly people is African American women over the age of seventy-five, followed by Hispanic women age seventy-five and older.

Table 6.1
Percentage of Poor and Near-Poor Elderly, by Age, Sex, and Race or
Ethnicity, 1990

Sex and Age	White Poor	White Near Poor	Black Poor	Black Near Poor	Hispanics[a] Poor	Hispanics[a] Near Poor	Total Poor	Total Near Poor
Both sexes								
65–74	7.4	4.9	29.6	11.0	20.6	10.4	9.7	5.4
75 and older	13.8	8.6	40.6	11.9	26.2	12.4	16.0	8.9
Male								
65–74	4.5	4.0	24.6	10.1	18.0	8.0	6.4	4.7
75 and older	7.8	4.5	34.4	12.0	20.1	9.1	9.9	6.0
Female								
65–74	10.2	5.6	33.6	11.7	22.7	12.3	12.3	6.1
75 and older	17.3	10.5	43.9	11.9	30.1	14.4	19.5	10.7

Source: U. S. General Accounting Office (1992).
[a] Hispanics may be of any race.

Four factors contribute to the risk of poverty for both men and women in older life: living longer, being widowed, living alone, or working in the secondary sector of the labor market. Yet each of these four factors is more likely to occur in women's lives (Gonyea 1994). Men typically do not bury their spouses, nor are they forced to live alone. For example, even at age eighty-five, less than one-quarter of all men live alone (U.S. Bureau of the Census 1992a), while women age seventy-five and older are likely to be widows (64%) and the majority (52%) live alone (U.S. Bureau of the Census 1994). What's more, for women age eighty-five and older living alone, the poverty rate is 32 percent—more than twice the rate for other women and men in this age group (15.2%; see Radner 1993).

Health

Historically, the image of very old people has been one of frailty. Yet, as Camacho et al. (1993) note, whereas "this is an accurate picture for some of the oldest-old, we know that there are many others who are able to maintain a high level of function at this age." Indeed, a growing number of researchers are exploring the phenomenon of "robust aging" among the oldest old (Harris et al. 1989; Garfein and Herzog 1995). The probability of having multiple chronic illnesses does, however, increase dramatically with age. Once again, the evidence shows men to be at an advantage. Although older men are more likely to experience fatal acute illnesses, older women are more likely to have chronic illnesses. Among those eighty years and older, 70 percent of women and 53 percent of men had two or more of the following conditions: arthritis, hypertension, cataracts, heart disease, varicose veins, diabetes, cancer, osteoporosis or hip fracture, and stroke. Similarly, the health disadvantage associated with minority status and lower social class in younger populations persists into late old age (Camacho et al. 1993), even in advanced welfare states such as Sweden (Thorsland and Lundberg 1994).

The need for personal assistance with everyday activities also increases sharply with advanced age. Whereas only 9 percent of those age sixty-five to seventy living in the community require assistance, this figure climbs to 45 percent of those eighty-five and older. (In each age group, women are more likely than men to require help, and elderly African Americans require more assistance than elderly whites.) By age eighty-five, if those in nursing homes are included, almost two-thirds of the age group are functionally dependent. Thus, the issue of long-term care dominates almost any discussion about the oldest old. It is especially relevant for older women, who, if they are not the recipients of long-term care, are likely to be the caregivers for someone who is. More than one-third of functionally dependent men age eighty-five and over live with and are primarily cared for by their wives. However, only 4 percent of their female counterparts live with their husbands.

Age-Based Programs and the Oldest Old

Because of the factors described above, the differential importance of public policy allocations for the oldest old, as compared to the young old, cannot be overstated. Social Security benefits constitute 71 percent of total income among poor elders, in contrast to only 31 percent among nonpoor elders (U.S. General Accounting Office 1992). Despite the higher utilization rates by the oldest old, Medicare provides the same benefits and imposes the same premium, copayment, and deductible charges on all enrollees. Moreover, only 65 percent of the oldest old hold supplemental private policies, compared to 74 percent of the young old (National Center for Health Statistics 1991). Most startling are data showing that elders with more functional limitations are less likely to hold supplemental policies than those with fewer limitations (U.S. Bureau of the Census 1986). This malalignment of both public and private coverage among different older populations accounts in large part for those age eighty-five and older facing out-of-pocket expenditures of $3,630 per capita, in comparison to only $1,430 for those sixty-five to sixty-nine (U.S. Bureau of the Census 1992b). Despite the presence (and cost) of Medicare, data from the National Medical Expenditure Survey show Medicare paying just over half (53%) of the health care expenses of elderly poor persons—who are disproportionately the oldest old. The means-tested Medicaid program offers additional support to poor elderly persons, most notably in paying their premiums and in being the dominant public payer for institutional long-term care. In 1989, approximately $48 billion was spent on nursing home care; just over half was paid for privately, and slightly under half was paid for by Medicaid (Short et al., 1992).

Riley, Kahn, and Forner (1994) offer the concept of "a structural lag" as a framework for understanding the mismatch between rapidly changing human lives, especially the phenomenon of longer and healthier lives, and social institutions. This concept is instructive in assessing the fit between population dynamics and policy design. One of the basic assumptions at the enactment of the Social Security program is no longer true: that only a small percentage of Americans would survive to old age to collect benefits and that those who did would receive benefits for only a brief period of time. Similarly, when Medicare was introduced in 1965, little attention was focused on demographic implications of the oldest old. Nor was it originally envisioned that Medicaid, a program designed to finance acute health care for low-income people of all ages, would become the primary third-party payer for nursing home care for a large segment of the elderly population.

Neugarten (1974), the pioneer in noting the heterogeneity of the aging population, created the labels *the young old* and *the old old* to emphasize that chronological age was increasingly becoming an inaccurate marker for one's health, economic, and social status. A decade later, Binstock (1985, 425) warned that Neugarten's attempt to break down age-based stereotypes was being substantially distorted: "Instead of confronting the issue of whether need rather than age is a relevant basis for structuring certain social policies, many policy analysts and public officials are fudging the issue. They consider policy options that would simply substitute age 75 (and other old ages) for a variety of younger ages now used as crude markers to approximate those within the older population who may need collective assistance."

As the evidence presented in this chapter suggests, well-being in advanced old age is shaped by economics, health, living arrangements, and social supports. Indeed, these factors are interrelated. As Hudson (1994, 745) stresses, "economic security is increasingly about adequate health and sickness coverage against potentially severe and unpredictable incapacities associated with advanced old age," just those areas where public policy protection has been weakest. Similarly, the risk of institutionalization is about social supports, especially the availability of family. The current cohort of the oldest old has fewer children than their earlier counterparts, and even when children are present, they are likely to be in their sixties or older and facing some functional impairment themselves. It is primarily the gender difference in survival that affects family structure and increases women's risk of nursing home placement. Raising the marker for age-based programs to seventy-five years addresses neither the diversity among the oldest old nor the question of need. Rather, it would only reinforce the stereotyping of the oldest old as a frail and marginal population.

Long-Term Care and the Oldest Old

Given these large national expenditures on behalf of elderly people, it is not surprising that age-based programs are receiving greater public scrutiny. Congressional proposals to reduce the size of the federal deficit or to balance the federal budget have increasingly focused on the restructuring of entitlements to older Americans by such practices as means testing, reducing Medicare coverage, and raising the age and increasing taxation of Social Security benefits (Torres-Gil and Puccinelli 1994; Kingson 1994). Despite considerable differences between those on the political right and left on the issue of age-based entitlements, there are two shared beliefs (Hudson 1994): that a growing number of elders are in reasonable economic circumstances and that a considerable number of elders have needs that are not being met. However, liberal advocates typically propose that the best solution is to make new or extended benefits available to the disadvantaged groups—older women, older people of color, and older people with low incomes. Conservative advocates, in contrast, argue for stricter targeting of benefits, typically through means tests, to significantly reduce the number of older people currently receiving benefits and, thereby, reaching the "truly needy." Yet, for both sides, the central question is the same: How do we reshape age-based policies to respond to the new demographic, health, and economic realities of the aging population?

Public debate about age-based programs often centers on the issue of long-term care, particularly concerns about the future level of need for such services and the ability of individuals to pay for this care. These are extraordinarily difficult questions to answer. The need for formal long-term care services is affected by not only the growing numbers of the oldest old but also their level of active life expectancy (the number of years a person can expect to live free of serious disability). The degree to which future cohorts of the oldest old will be healthier than previous cohorts remains unknown. Some researchers argue that better lifestyles and health habits as well as improved medical treatments are contributing to a phenomenon of "compressed morbidity" (Fries 1989; Manton and Stallard 1991; Manton, Corder, and Stallard 1993), while others suggest that more people may live long enough to suffer from debilitating conditions such as dementia (Evans, Funkenstein, and Albert 1989). Yet, more than one's physical health affects the need for long-term care. Even if we postpone the age of death, "we may also be postponing the period of intense service need until even later in the life cycle, when fewer financial and/or family resources may be available" (Soldo and Manton 1985, 314).

Determining elders' ability to pay for their own long-term care is also a difficult task, but some inferences can be made. For example, in one study based on computer simulations of the 1989 Long-Term Care Survey, Sloan and Shayne (1993) found that 19 percent of individuals in the community were already on Medicaid and 59 percent of the disabled elders not on Medicaid would have qualified for Medicaid immediately on nursing home entry. These findings are typical, and there is no reason to assume that future cohorts of the oldest old will be better able to afford long-term care. The relative increase in retirement benefits in recent decades may not continue in the long run. Pension coverage has declined in recent years because of the loss of jobs in the manufacturing sector and the growth of jobs in the service sector. Almost 80 percent of employed Americans now work in the service sector in jobs that typically offer low wages and few or no insurance or retirement benefits; by the year 2000, it is projected, this figure will reach 92 percent (Schuping 1992). The scheduled increase in Social Security retirement age also means that benefits paid to future retirees at any specific age will decline. Moreover, with the continued extension of the period beyond retirement (due to greater life expectancy), the oldest old will have to contend with the inflationary decline in value of their pensions. Most pension plans are not fully indexed with inflation and lose real value with each passing year. For many of the oldest old, the dilemma will be how to meet increasing health care costs on a declining income.

The U.S. system of long-term care is firmly planted in a residualist tradition, wherein government provides benefits only when the family and market sources have failed. There is a growing public sentiment, however, that families should not be forced to face impoverishment as a result of long-term care costs and that a financing mechanism that provides an alternative to means-tested Medicaid is needed. Since the mid-1980s, there has been considerable growth in the number of private insurance companies offering long-term care insurance. Yet, from a public policy perspective, private insurance is unlikely to provide adequate funding for long-term care. Only 3 percent of Americans have long-term care insurance. From the consumer's perspective, these private policies have a number of disadvantages: the cost of the policies is very high, annual premiums typically ranging from $2,600 to $4,000; many people are excluded from purchasing policies because of preexisting physical conditions or mental disorders; most policies do not adequately cover home care and other noninstitutional care; and people with long-lasting but medically stable conditions (for example, Alzheimer's disease) find it difficult to qualify for benefits. Nor is the affordability of privately marketed long-term care insurance likely to change significantly in the future (Reif 1989). Computer simulations suggest that even by the year 2030 only 10 percent of elderly persons will be able to purchase private long-term care insurance at a cost of less than 5 percent of their total income (Zedlewski and McBride 1992).

As an alternative to either public assistance Medicaid or the private market, the United States could offer families more complete protection against the catastrophic costs of long-term care by adopting a public insurance model. Despite our nation's historical residualistic philosophy, social insurance models have been successfully implemented to avert two other potential economic catastrophes confronted by families. Social Security represents a social insurance approach to protect families from impoverishment in old age caused by inadequate retirement income and savings. Similarly, Medicare protects individuals against poverty caused by lack of acute medical care coverage in old age. A growing number of policy analysts are advocating the adoption of a social insurance approach to protect families from a third potential economic catastrophe, the costs of long-term care (Brody 1987; Hudson 1994). In fact, Sloan and Shayne (1993, 596) suggest that "the spousal impoverishment provision of the Medicare Catastrophic Coverage Act of 1988 pushed the nation further in the direction of universal long-term care financing, perhaps inadvertently." Although the intent of Congress in the passage of this legislation was to make it more difficult for families to transfer assets in order to qualify for Medicaid in a nursing home, it in fact essentially eliminated the need for married disabled spouses to transfer assets if they believed their spouses would survive them and remain in the community.

A clear advantage of a compulsory and universal public insurance model for protection against the costs of long-term care is that it allows the creation of large risk pools. By doing so, it avoids the adverse selection problem found in private market insurance, which ultimately drives cost upward and makes policies unaffordable to most potential consumers. Yet, only if demand is strong enough will public long-term care insurance be considered an option. Perhaps the best prospect for resolving the challenges for developing and financing a public insurance model for long-term care lies in the building of coalitions of advocates for the aging and advocates for the disabled. Such a strategy suggests that the social insurance must be functionally based and not population centered. Although the presence of chronic illness and disabilities is positively correlated with age, aging does not equal disability. In fact, of household members with a chronic disability in need of care, 12 percent are children under the age of twenty, 44 percent are adults ages twenty to fifty-nine, and 44 percent are individuals age sixty and older (Center for Vulnerable Populations 1992). In the recent national debate on health care reform, both the McDermott/Wellstone single-payer plan and President Clinton's health care plan included long-term care services for individuals of all ages based on a beneficiary's need for assistance in performing activities of daily life, severe cognitive or mental impairment, or profound mental retardation. Despite the failure of these legislative proposals to move forward, they have clearly established the principle that public insurance for long-term care will be based on need-for-service criteria rather than age-based criteria (Binstock 1994).

Conclusion

The importance of age-based programs for the oldest old is beyond dispute. Eighty-five percent of people age eighty-five and older report receiving at least half of their income from Social Security, and virtually all elderly persons gain access to health care coverage (hospital and physician services) through Medicare. To a large extent, the success of these programs lies in the decision to design them based on social insurance principles. Inherent in both programs is the concept of providing universal protection to older citizens for the loss of income in old age through compulsory participation in order to allow the pooling of resources and the sharing of risk. It has long been recognized that universal programs avoid the stigmatization and stereotyping that occurs with means-tested programs. Moreover, the decision to establish these programs as age based makes sense in that, for the majority of Americans, income and access to health care insurance are connected to employment.

While these age-based programs have improved the aggregate well-being of older people, they do not adequately address the differences that exist within the aging population, including those of advanced old age. Clearly, a significant proportion of the oldest old are vulnerable. Relative to the young old, the oldest old are poorer and in worse physical health. Even among these "elite survivors," inequalities by gender, race, and social class exist (Thorsland and Lundberg 1994; Crystal and Shea 1990). These inequalities are derived from the fact that, although the United States does a better job than other industrialized countries in maintaining preretirement income in old age, it has one of the least egalitarian systems of income distribution before retirement (Myles 1988). The accumulated effects of early and midlife experiences—labor force opportunities, health behaviors, living conditions, and social supports—influence the economic and health circumstances individuals face in old age. For example, the assumption that people before age sixty-five have employment-based health insurance coverage is simply incorrect for a growing number (especially women and people of color) working in the secondary or contingent workforce. Further, there is evidence that income disparities not only are maintained but also are amplified across the life course (Crystal and Shea 1990). The link between economics and health is particularly relevant for the oldest old. Despite their diversity, by age eighty-five, almost two-thirds of this group are functionally dependent, and out-of-pocket health care expenses have an impact on poor people. One of the greatest threats to the economic security of the oldest old remains long-term care expenses. In the current political climate, however, proposing a particularistic reform for elderly people would serve only to fuel the fires of the "generational equity" debate. In fact, the catastrophic cost associated with long-term care is not just an aging issue. Age is correlated with, but not defined by, disability. More than half the people with chronic disabilities living in the community are under the age of sixty-five, and almost all Americans (97%)—regardless of race, gender, or class—are unprotected against the catastrophic health care costs associated with chronic illnesses. While the oldest old have much to gain, perhaps politically the best way to achieve social insurance against the catastrophic costs of long-term care services is through a functionally based, and not an age-based, program.

References

Barer, B. 1994. Men and Women Aging Differently. *International Journal of Aging and Human Development* 38:29–40.

Binstock, R. 1985. The Oldest Old: A Fresh Perspective or Compassionate Ageism Revisited? *Milbank Quarterly* 63:420–51.

———. 1994. Changing Criteria in Old-Age Programs: The Introduction of Economic Status and Need for Services. *Gerontologist* 34:726–30.

Brody, S. 1987. Strategic Planning: The Catastrophic Approach. *Gerontologist* 27:131–38.

Callahan, D. 1987. *Setting Limits: Medical Goals in an Aging Society.* New York: Simon and Schuster.

Camacho, T., W. Strawbridge, R. Cohen, and G. Kaplan. 1993. Functional Ability in the Oldest Old. *Journal of Aging and Health* 5:439–54.

Center for Vulnerable Populations. 1992. *Familiar Faces—The Status of America's Vulnerable Populations: A Chartbook.* Portland, Maine: Center for Health Policy Development.

Crystal, S., and D. Shea. 1990. Cumulative Advantage, Cumulative Disadvantage, and Inequality among Elderly People. *Gerontologist* 30:437–43.

Evans, D., H. Funkenstein, and M. Albert. 1989. Prevalence of Alzheimer's Disease in a Community Population of Older Persons. *Journal of the American Medical Association* 262:2551–56.

Fries, J. 1989. The Compression of Morbidity: Near or Far? *Milbank Quarterly* 67:208–32.

Garfein, A., and A. Herzog. 1995. Robust Aging among the Young-Old, Old-Old, and Oldest-Old. *Journal of Gerontology: Social Sciences* 50b:s77–87.

Gonyea, J. 1994. Making Gender Visible in Public Policy. In E. Thompson Jr., ed., *Older Men's Lives.* Thousand Oaks, Calif.: Sage.

Harris, C. 1978. *Fact Book on Aging*. Washington, D.C.: National Council on Aging.

Harris, T., M. Kovar, R. Suzman, J. Kleinman, and J. Feldman. 1989. Longitudinal Study of Physical Ability in the Oldest-Old. *American Journal of Public Health* 79:698–702.

Hudson, R. 1978. The "Graying" of the Federal Budget and Its Consequences for Old Age Policy. *Gerontologist* 18:428–40.

———. 1994. A Contingency-Based Approach for Assessing Policies on Aging. *Gerontologist* 34:743–48.

Kingson, E. 1994. Testing the Boundaries of Universality: What's Mean? What's Not? *Gerontologist* 34:736–42.

Longino, C., Jr. 1988. A Population Profile of Very Old Men and Women in the United States. *Sociology Quarterly* 29:559–64.

Manton, K., L. Corder, and E. Stallard. 1993. Estimates of Change in Chronic Disability and Institutional Incidence and Prevalence Rates in the U.S. Elderly Population from 1982, 1984, and 1989. *Journal of Gerontology: Social Sciences* 48:s153–66.

Manton, K., and E. Stallard. 1991. Cross-Sectional Estimates of Active Life Expectancy for the U.S. Elderly and Oldest-Old Populations. *Journal of Gerontology: Social Sciences* 46:s170–82.

Myles, J. 1988. Postwar Capitalism and the Extension of Social Security into the Retirement Wage. In M. Weir, A. Orloff, and T. Skocpol, eds., *The Politics of Social Policy in the United States*. Princeton: Princeton University Press.

National Center for Health Statistics 1991. *Health United States, 1990*. Hyattsville, Md.: Public Health Service.

Neugarten, B. 1974. Age Groups in American Society and the Rise of the Young-Old. In F. Eisele, ed., *Political Consequences of Aging*. Philadelphia: American Academy of Political and Social Sciences.

Radner, D. 1993. Economic Well-Being of the Old Old: Family Unit Income and Household Wealth. *Social Security Bulletin* 56:3–19.

Reif, L. 1989. Epilogue: The Future. In S. Bould, B. Sandborn, and L. Reif, eds., *Eighty- Five Plus: The Oldest Old*. Belmont, Calif.: Wadsworth.

Riley, M., R. Kahn, and A. Forner, eds. 1994. *Age and Structural Lag*. New York: Wiley.

Robertson, A. 1991. The Politics of Alzheimer's Disease: A Case Study in Apocalyptic Demography. In M. Minkler and C. Estes, eds., *Critical Perspectives on Aging: The Political and Moral Economy of Growing Old*. New York: Baywood.

Schuping, J. 1992. Industry-at-Large: Information Integration—Key to Business Success. *Electronic News* 38:11–12.

Short, P., P. Kemper, L. Cornelius, and D. Walden. 1992. Public and Private Responsibility for Financing Nursing Home Care: The Effect of Medicaid Asset Spend-down. *Milbank Quarterly* 70:277–98.

Sloan, F., and M. Shayne. 1993. Long-Term Care and Impoverishment of the Elderly. *Milbank Quarterly* 71:575–99.

Soldo, B., and K. Manton. 1985. Health Status and Service Needs of the Oldest Old: Current Patterns and Future Trends. *Milbank Quarterly* 63:286–319.

Suzman, R., and M. Riley. 1985. Introducing the "Oldest-Old." *Milbank Quarterly* 63:177–86.

Thompson, E., Jr. 1994. Older Men as Invisible Men in Contemporary Society. In E. Thompson Jr., ed., *Older Men's Lives*. Thousand Oaks, Calif.: Sage.

Thorsland, M., and O. Lundberg. 1994. Health and Inequalities among the Oldest Old. *Journal of Aging and Health* 6:51–69.

Torres-Gil, F., and M. Puccinelli. 1994. Mainstreaming Gerontology in the Policy Arena. *Gerontologist* 34:749–52.

Treas, J., and V. Bengtson. 1982. The Demography of Mid- and Late-Life Transitions. *Annals of the American Academy of Political and Social Science* 464:11–21.

U.S. Bureau of the Census. 1986. *Disability, Functional Limitation, and Health Insurance Coverage.* Current Population Reports, Series P-70, No. 8. Washington, D.C.: Government Printing Office.

———. 1992a. *Population Projections of the United States, by Age, Sex, Race, and Hispanic Origin.* Current Population Reports, Series P-25, No. 1092. Washington, D.C.: Government Printing Office.

———. 1992b. *Sixty-Five Plus in America.* Current Population Reports, Series P-23, No. 178. Washington, D.C.: Government Printing Office.

———. 1994. Marital Status of the Population, by Sex and Age, 1993. *Statistical Abstract of the United States,* 114th ed. Washington, D.C.: Government Printing Office.

U.S. General Accounting Office. 1992. *Elderly Americans: Health, Housing, and Nutrition Gaps between the Poor and Nonpoor.* GAO/pemd-92-29. Washington, D.C.: Government Printing Office.

Zedlewski, S., and T. McBride. 1992. The Changing Profile of the Elderly: Effects on Future Long-Term Care Needs and Financing. *Milbank Quarterly* 70:247–76.

7

The Young Old, Productive Aging, and Public Policy

ROBERT MORRIS and FRANCIS G. CARO

Both public policy and employer policy have encouraged the development of a large pool of individuals, not members of the full-time workforce, called the near old (set somewhat arbitrarily at age fifty-five through sixty-four) and the young old (age sixty-five through seventy-four). Key questions raised by this development include, How can society draw more effectively on this group to meet community service needs? How can new opportunities be created for older people through both paid employment and voluntarist activities? And how can projects be designed and implemented to test creative and low-cost ways of engaging older people as volunteers in addressing community needs? In addition to referencing the considerable body of literature addressing retirement and volunteering, this chapter draws especially on the findings of the Commonwealth Fund's Productive Aging Study (PAS), a survey of a representative national sample of 2,999 non-institutionalized persons age fifty-five and older (Caro and Bass 1992).

The Trend toward Early Retirement

A major economic achievement of the industrialized countries has been the development of pension programs that provide substantial long-term retirement income. Largely as a result of Social Security and a growing economy, poverty levels among old people in the United

States declined between 1959 and 1992 by a factor of three, and median incomes of families headed by older people (as measured in inflation-adjusted 1989 dollars) increased from $13,620 in 1965 to $22,806 in 1989. Social Security is the major contributor to these improvements, constituting 41 percent of aggregate income among all aged households in 1991. Returns on assets, private pensions, and earnings followed in importance, and these sources are relatively more important for the young old than for the old old.

These economic improvements have been accompanied by both earlier retirement ages among older Americans and improved morbidity and mortality trends. The retirement age among older men has (until very recently) fallen dramatically. In 1950, 87 percent of men age fifty-five through sixty-four and 46 percent of men age sixty-five and older participated in the labor market, compared to 67 percent and 16 percent, respectively, in 1991. Mortality data show that life expectancy increased between 1970 and 1985: for white males it increased 13.0–14.6 years, and for white females it increased 16.9–18.7 years (Manton 1990). The review by Manton, Stallard, and Corder (1995) of the National Long-Term Care Study data also shows consistent declines in morbidity and disability rates among emerging cohorts of older Americans.

A number of factors have been at work in the trend toward earlier retirement. There is, however, disagreement concerning the relative importance of each. Observers agree that the introduction of the early retirement option under Social Security and the liberalizations in Social Security benefits in recent years have played a major role. Quinn, Burkhauser, and Myers (1990) report that studies modeling the retirement decision have found Social Security and private pension availability to have the greatest impact on the decision to retire.

Yet, the situations of those taking advantage of these provisions may vary considerably, there being most notably an important distinction between those who leave the labor force in good health and with favorable retirement income prospects and those whose health and future income status are more marginal (Kingson 1979; Crown 1990). Recent evidence suggests movement in the former direction, and among the near old and the young old in the PAS sample who were unemployed, 64 percent and 63 percent, respectively, reported themselves to be in excellent or good health. In addition to early retirees, there are, as well, growing numbers of older part-time workers. Indeed, those taking Social Security benefits before age sixty-five are more likely to work part-time or to be self-employed than are older retirees (Quinn, Burkhauser, and Myers 1990; Hudson and Kingson forthcoming). The trend toward early retirement brings with it a number of complex issues.

Access to Employment

The early departure of older people from the workforce has often been interpreted positively. That society has been able to provide economic security to large numbers of older persons through public and private income-transfer programs is itself a historic development. Increases in productivity gains have also made this wealth creation possible in the absence of large numbers of able-bodied older workers. And, of course, retirement has been a positive force in precluding conflicts between younger and older workers, allowing younger people to hold jobs and be promoted earlier than would otherwise be the case.

Despite both widespread preferences to retire and the increased ability to do so, there remain serious concerns for many older people who find themselves unemployed. By no means are all labor force withdrawals voluntary, many being for reasons of ill health or structural unemployment in different geographic settings and, most recently, as the result of the brutal downsizing of many American corporations, often accomplished through layoffs rather than early retirement incentives. Layoffs trigger premature departure of the near old and the young old from the labor force; of the 46 percent of the near old in the PAS sample who were not working, 20 percent reported that they were willing and able to work. Because older workers have greater difficulty in finding replacement jobs than do younger workers and may also have greater difficulty in changing fields (O'Reilly and Caro 1995), new opportunities are needed for workforce participation. Such initiatives might include a tailored analysis of local labor markets, career counseling, retraining, and placement services (Caro and Morris 1992).

There are serious shortcomings in contemporary public policies directed toward these issues. The Job Training Partnership Act (JTPA) includes a modest provision for older workers, but a means test is imposed on workers over age fifty-five, and funding under the act is limited. The Older Americans Act Title V program is funded to the tune of some $300 million, but its application is limited to low-income individuals over age fifty-five whose employment prospects are deemed "poor." Enforcement of the Age Discrimination in Employment Act has been uneven over the years, and discrimination based on negative attitudes toward older workers continues (Wineman 1990). A review of age discrimination cases filed with the Massachusetts Commission against Discrimination in 1989 found that only 15 percent had an outcome favorable to the worker, and those older workers with complaints specifically about hiring practices fared even worse (Caro and Motika 1992).

Despite these combinations of "push and pull" forces propelling and compelling older workers out of the labor force, the economy still contains many niches in which there are labor shortages and in which older workers could be usefully employed. Of particular interest here are positions for which older workers may be particularly well qualified because the positions call for experience, skill in working with others, skill in dealing with the public, reliability, and accuracy rather than speed. The Commonwealth Fund (1993) reports on a number of successful corporate experiments that drew on the near old and the young old as niche employees. Among these is the Days Inn Corporation's hiring of older people as telephone reservation agents. Riekse (1991) offers another example, an older worker retraining program at Grand Rapids (Michigan) Community College that is supported by an automobile manufacturer who hires older people to finish wooden dashboards for luxury cars. An analysis of specific labor markets is needed to identify more opportunities for the young old to reenter the labor market as niche employees.

Public policy needs to better ensure that access to employment opportunities is independent of age. Advancing age by itself should not prevent interested and qualified individuals from obtaining and retaining jobs. At the very least, public policy to support productive paid work for the near old and the young old should (1) strengthen the enforcement provisions under the Age Discrimination in Employment Act, (2) reduce the earnings test under Social Security so that the tax on earnings is comparable to income tax rates and raise the earnings limit, (3) support stronger comprehensive retraining and job placement programs for the near old, and (4) support research to identify labor market niches that could be filled effectively by older workers.

The Needs of Family Caregivers

Older people make substantial unpaid contributions within the family in both caring for grandchildren and providing long-term care. The

PAS findings document the extent of these efforts. In the PAS sample, 12 percent of the near old and 10 percent of the young old were providing twenty hours a week or more in caring for grandchildren; 5 percent of the near old and the young old were caring for the sick and disabled for twenty or more hours per week. Public policy has failed to acknowledge the needs of some of those who make the major productive contributions within the family.

Of particular concern are older women who have a limited history of paid employment because they were extensively involved in a succession of child care and long-term care roles through much of their adult lives (Brody 1990). These women enter old age without qualifying for private pensions and lack an adequate retirement base in social insurance.

A variety of public policy options are available to recognize those who make extraordinary productive contributions within the family. One possibility is to make cash payments to certain family members for providing extensive child care or long-term care. Precedents exist for paying those who provide long-term care to community-residing relatives, but cash payment programs are controversial (Keigher and Stone 1994). At a minimum, those who are engaged in extensive care of grandchildren or extensive informal long-term care should receive Social Security earning credits. Special employment opportunities in child care or home care might also be developed for informal caregivers when their obligations within the family lessen or come to an end. Federal job training programs for displaced homemakers provide a precedent for programs to assist older women who seek a transition from extensive family responsibilities to paid employment. Whatever the mechanism, public policies are particularly needed to ensure adequate income in old age for those who lack both private pensions and Social Security earning credits because of their careers in providing unpaid care within the family.

The Community Service Crisis

Ironically, our national economic policies ensure less than full participation of able people in the workforce, yet the community service sector suffers from neglect. We are confronted with serious shortages in the resources needed to address community problems. The strains are particularly evident at the level of local government, where public services touch concretely on the lives of people. We hear, for example, about strains on budgets for schools, public safety, libraries, and recreation programs.

The resource deficiencies are particularly visible in the human services, whether they are offered by public or private agencies. The public/private distinction matters little, since both rely heavily on public funding (Smith and Lipsky 1993). Whether they serve young people or old people, providers of subsidized services struggle constantly with resource constraints. Public funds have been cut, and private fundraising rarely is a source of adequate replacement funds. Even the health sector, which for many years enjoyed favored status, is now subject to strong pressures to cut costs.

Programs that depend on public funds are squeezed by rising costs and growing public resistance to tax increases. The economic pressures that limit the tax resources available to community services run deep and are long-standing. They are probably influenced by a gradual decline in per capita productivity in the United States since the early 1970s (Chen 1994). Problems of financing are particularly serious for labor-intensive services. Education, police work, social services, and health programs are all inherently highly labor-intensive. Rapid increases in health insurance costs have increased financial burdens for employers who offer standard fringe benefit packages to employees. In the human service field, the potential for substituting technology for people is modest. Programs everywhere are under pressure to reduce their personnel costs. Increasingly, programs must be receptive to strategies that reduce their reliance on fully benefited personnel who receive market wages.

The consequences of weak service systems are serious. The unprecedented involvement of children in violent crime illustrates the inadequacies of our social services in the face of persistent poverty, racial discrimination, and serious weaknesses in nuclear families. At the other end of the age spectrum, frail, confused older people who live alone are often left to manage with only sketchy service supports.

Productive Contributions through Volunteering

Our major question is how the near old and the young old who are retired and economically secure can be more effectively engaged in addressing the nation's crisis in community services (Morris and Caro forthcoming). In the 1880s, Simon Patten, an American sociologist-cum-economist, predicted an era of expanded leisure following technological innovations that would confront society with new ethical and moral issues about how such mass leisure would be used (Fox 1967). What Patten did not anticipate, however, was a society that despite great private wealth did not provide adequate financial resources for conventional solutions for its community service needs. However, an early observer, Alexis de Tocqueville (Tocqueville 1955) was impressed with this nation's efforts to address community needs through the organized efforts of volunteers.

Can we find more effective ways to engage healthy, economically secure near-old and young-old people as volunteers to address the nation's unmet community service needs? These groups are already making useful contributions, but the potential for greater contributions is substantial. Data from PAS illustrate the point. Approximately 30 percent of the near old and the young old who were not working were volunteers. However, the typical volunteering effort was modest; the median number of volunteer hours reported was four hours a week. A notable minority were very active: 29 percent and 25 percent, respectively, of near-old and young-old volunteers contributed twenty or more hours per week.

The near old and the young old are often also involved in providing important informal help in their families and neighborhoods. Approximately 53 percent of the near old and 44 percent of the young old were involved in helping children or grandchildren, and 36 percent of the near old and 33 percent of the young old were engaged in helping sick or disabled people. In a substantial proportion of cases, the number of hours a week of these unpaid productive activities is impressive. For 29 percent and 25 percent of near-old and young-old persons, respectively, the weekly hours of volunteering, helping children or grandchildren, and helping the sick or disabled totaled twenty hours or more.

The fact that many are already engaged in formal and informal help to their families and communities is encouraging but invites the question whether substantially more productive activity is possible. The PAS provides evidence that many who do not volunteer could do so. Among nonvolunteers, 24 percent and 17 percent of near-old and young-old persons, respectively, indicated that they were both willing and able to volunteer. Roughly, for every two in these age groups who volunteer, another respondent indicated receptivity to volunteering.

Enhancing Volunteer Activities

We suspect that a substantial revitalization of volunteering will occur only if relationships between volunteers and paid personnel are redefined. Most community services in the United States originated as strictly volunteer efforts (Ellis and Noyes 1990). Only when the demand for services increased and the supply of volunteers was insufficient were paid personnel introduced. The early paid staff were often coordinators of volunteers. With the hiring of full-time personnel came emphasis on the expertise that paid professionals could bring; because volunteers were regarded as amateurs, they were often devalued. In this way, paid personnel have come to dominate most community service organizations, and volunteers have been relegated to marginal duties. In part, the modest contributions of volunteers in many organizations may be a self-fulfilling prophecy. Typically, because they are not trusted to carry out more important work, volunteers are given light responsibilities requiring little training or supervision. However, many capable individuals are reluctant to make a substantial commitment to volunteering because the assignments open to them are not challenging. Several questions follow from this. To what extent can community service organizations assign more challenging responsibilities to volunteers? To what extent will older people respond to opportunities to make more significant contributions as volunteers? Under what circumstances can community services be restructured so that some significant responsibilities are shifted from paid personnel to volunteers?

A number of efforts involving older volunteers have proved successful. Three federal Great Society programs for older volunteers are now well established (Butler 1992). The Retired Senior Volunteer Program (RSVP) engages older people as volunteers in a variety of roles developed by local sponsors. However, the demands on RSVP volunteers tend to be modest with respect to both the time commitments asked of them and the duties assigned. The Senior Companion program and the Foster Grandparent program fall in the gray area between volunteer and employment programs. In both cases, older people serve twenty hours a week and receive a modest stipend. Eligibility is limited to those who pass a means test. These programs certainly demonstrate that older people can be recruited as stipended volunteers and can be placed successfully in a variety of community settings. However, the scope of these programs is limited by modest levels of federal funding. They do not provide sufficient opportunities for the many low-income elderly people who would be interested in participating, and no similar opportunities for extensive volunteering are provided for the large group of middle-income early retirees.

Precedents can also be found for viable community services staffed by volunteers. The conspicuous examples that can be readily identified in many smaller communities are volunteer fire department and ambulance services. In a serious effort to compare professional and volunteer fire departments, Brudney and Duncombe (1992) found professional units to be superior; nevertheless, the performance of the volunteer units tended to be credible. Yet, a number of major obstacles must be addressed if community services are to be revitalized through an infusion of older volunteers.

Conflict between Paid Personnel and Volunteers

Paid personnel can view volunteers as economic competitors. Volunteers can undermine the economic leverage of paid personnel. In organizations that seek cooperative relationships between volunteers and paid personnel, volunteer assignments must be structured in ways that are sensitive to the economic interests of paid personnel. One important possibility is to assign volunteers to clearly defined duties that organizations cannot afford to have staffed by paid personnel. Volunteers are likely to be accepted by paid workers when the organizational choice is volunteer staffing or no service at all. Another possibility is contracting with volunteer organizations. Brudney (1990) recommends this approach for public agencies. Some public agencies may find it easier to delegate certain responsibilities to volunteers who are associated with a separate organization than to integrate volunteers and paid staff members internally.

Significant Volunteer Assignments

Suitable assignments are needed. We propose that organizations assign greater responsibilities to volunteers; we also predict that capable older people can be found who will welcome the challenge. The limits of what older volunteers can contribute on a continuing basis will be known only when organizations risk assigning important responsibilities to volunteers. Realism is needed in structuring responsibilities. Older volunteers, for example, are not likely to take on physically demanding assignments, but they are likely to be interested in assignments in which they are asked to provide information to the public.

Older volunteers are not likely to be willing to work forty hours a week but may be attracted to assignments that ask for a commitment of two days a week.

Investment in Volunteers

While volunteers can be attractive resources, they are not free. If volunteers are to make significant contributions, substantial organizational investment is required in structuring assignments, recruitment, screening, training, supervision, and recognition. For volunteers making significant time commitments, a stipend may be important even if the payment level is modest.

Cost-Benefit Analysis

We propose the use of older volunteers in significant assignments as a mechanism for enabling communities to make more effective use of limited financial resources. However, cost-benefit analysis is essential to ensure that the strategy of using older volunteers is used only in instances in which it yields results superior to those achieved with conventional staffing.

AmeriCorps Elder Leadership Program

We have launched an initiative to test the approach in one area of application—the delivery of community services to older people in the Boston area. Councils on aging and home care corporations are publicly funded service brokers who are challenged to meet the growing demand for services with contracting public funds (Kent 1995). Within the framework of the federal AmeriCorps program, the elder leadership program recruits near-old and young-old people as stipended volunteers to serve as volunteer coordinators within local councils on aging and home care corporations. AmeriCorps members strengthen a variety of volunteer services such as telephone reassurance, medical escort, light chore services, and shopping for frail elders. Hard-pressed councils on aging already make extensive use of volunteers, recognize the need for greater volunteer productivity, and welcome the prospect of the addition of half-time, skilled, volunteer coordinators. In this instance, AmeriCorps will provide older members with a modest stipend and an affiliation with a significant national community-building effort.

Research and Demonstrations

A stimulus is needed to encourage community service organizations to experiment with more significant volunteer opportunities for near-old and young-old people. Within participating organizations, substantial effort will be required to overcome widespread skepticism about the willingness of older people to accept more significant volunteer responsibilities and about their ability to perform in more responsible positions. Groundwork will also have to be laid carefully to gain the support of paid personnel. Well-designed evaluation research will be needed to provide sound evidence regarding the effectiveness of the interventions.

We urge a classic demonstration effort in which substantial grant funds are made available to several centers to foster the development of specific initiatives. We envision that the centers will provide seed money to community service organizations to assist them in designing specific demonstrations and that they will also conduct evaluation research and disseminate the findings.

Conclusion

Paid and unpaid work by near-old and young-old people who are healthy is a major aspect of an aging society in the twenty-first century. The concept of continuing participation in the economic and public life of society regardless of age represents a major shift from the prevailing thinking in the 1930s, when the removal of older people from the full life of the society was encouraged. The 1930s laid the foundation for relatively generous provisions to retire from work. Yet, the aging of the population and the growing proportion of retirees in the total population provide an opportunity to address our current crisis in community problem solving.

References

Brody, E. 1990. *Women in the Middle: Their Parent Care Years.* New York: Springer.

Brudney, J. 1990. *Fostering Volunteer Programs in the Public Sector.* San Francisco: Jossey-Bass.

Brudney, J., and W. Duncombe. 1992. An Economic Evaluation of Paid, Volunteer, and Mixed Staffing Options for Public Services. *Public Administration Review* 52:474–81.

Butler, F. 1992. *Program Descriptions: Older American Volunteer Programs.* Reston, Va.: National Directors Association.

Caro, F., and S. Bass. 1992. *Patterns of Productive Activity among Older Americans.* Boston: Gerontology Institute, University of Massachusetts.

Caro, F., and R. Morris. 1992. Retraining Older Workers: An Emerging Economic Need. *Community College Journal* 63:22–26.

Caro, F., and S. Motika. 1992. *Age Discrimination in Employment: A Review of Cases Filed with the Massachusetts Commission against Discrimination.* Boston: Gerontology Institute, University of Massachusetts.

Chen, Y.-P. 1994. Equivalent Retirement Ages and Their Implications for Social Security and Medicare Financing. *Gerontologist* 34:731–35.

Commonwealth Fund. 1993. *The Untapped Resource.* New York.

Crown, W. 1990. Economic Trends, Politics, and Employment Policy for Older Workers. *Journal of Aging and Social Policy* 2:131–51.

Ellis, S., and K. Noyes. 1990. *By the People: A History of Americans as Volunteers.* San Francisco: Jossey-Bass.

Fox, D. 1967. *The Discovery of Abundance.* Ithaca: Cornell University Press.

Hudson, R., and E. Kingson. Forthcoming. The Emerging Social Security Agenda: Retirement Income, Labor Market, and Financing Issues. *Policy Studies Review.*

Keigher, S., and R. Stone. 1994. Toward an Equitable Universal Caregiver Policy: The Potential of Financial Supports for Family Caregivers. *Journal of Aging and Social Policy* 6:57–75.

Kent, K. 1995. *Running on Empty.* Boston: Gerontology Institute, University of Massachusetts.

Kingson, E. 1979. Men Who Leave the Workforce before Age Sixty-two: A Study of Advantaged and Disadvantaged Very Early Retirement. Ph.D. diss., University of Michigan.

Manton, K. 1990. Mortality and Morbidity. In R. Binstock and L. George, eds., *Handbook of Aging and the Social Sciences,* 3d ed. San Diego: Academic.

Manton, K., E. Stallard, and L. Corder. 1995. Changes in Morbidity and Chronic Disability in the U.S. Elderly Population: Evidence from the 1982, 1984, and 1989 National Long-Term Care Surveys. *Journal of Gerontology: Social Sciences* 50b:s194–204.

Morris, R., and F. Caro. Forthcoming. Changing Boundaries between Work, Retirement, and Volunteerism: Retiree Volunteers to Meet Social Needs. *Ageing International.*

O'Reilly, P., and F. Caro. 1994. Productive Aging: An Overview of the Literature. *Journal of Aging and Social Policy* 6:39–71.

Quinn, J., R. Burkhauser, and D. Myers. 1990. *Passing the Torch: The Influence of Economic Incentives on Work and Retirement.* Kalamazoo, Mich.: Upjohn Institute for Employment Research.

Riekse, R. 1991. *Reclaiming a National Treasure: Retraining Economically Vulnerable Older Persons for the Contemporary Workplace.* Grand Rapids, Mich.: Grand Rapids Community College.

Smith, S., and M. Lipsky. 1993. *Nonprofits for Hire: The Welfare State in the Age of Contracting*. Cambridge: Harvard University Press.

Tocqueville, A. 1955 (1831). *Democracy in America*. New York: Vintage.

Wineman, J. 1990. Services to Older and Retired Workers. In A. Monk, ed., *Handbook of Gerontological Services*. New York: Columbia University Press.

8

The Old, the Young,
and the Welfare State

PAUL ADAMS and GARY L. DOMINICK

Concern about the impact of population aging on the federal deficit has heightened a perception held by many of greedy elders enriching themselves at the expense of succeeding generations. In this view, low fertility and population aging produce spending cuts for children and families, as older adults mobilize to protect their own position while opposing spending for children (Preston 1984). *Business Week* asks, "Is there a relationship between the aging of the population and the current push to cut federal aid for education, school lunches, and the like, while keeping Social Security sacrosanct?" (Koretz 1995, 42).

There are, however, problems in framing relations between old and young as an unequal struggle between competing interest groups. First, there is no necessary connection between high spending for older adults and low spending for children. Programs for older adults do not compete directly with those for children any more than with other programs. In fact, segments of the business community are probably more likely to see Social Security and Medicare as competition than are child and family advocates. Quadagno (1990, 637) finds major support and funding for the coalition Americans for Generational Equity coming from "banks, insurance companies, defense contractors, and health care corporations."

Second, older Americans, though they are more likely than other age groups to vote and to support organizations that lobby against cuts in Social Security, include members of different classes with conflicting interests. As Heclo (1988, 393) says, "the elderly and their advocacy organizations are far from a self-conscious, monolithic force in pursuit of self-interested claims on the public budget. Nor should this fact be surprising, once we realize that 'the elderly' is really a category created by policy analysts, pension officials, and mechanical models of interest group politics."

Third, in high-income welfare states as a group, there is no pattern of high spending on elderly people producing low spending for children. In many, the growing proportion of elders and declining proportion of children have been associated with increased spending for children (Pampel and Adams 1992; Pampel 1994). There, the growing ratio of public pension beneficiaries to contributors, much higher than in the United States, has heightened awareness of the importance of child rearing as a contribution to society in general and to social security in particular. It has led to a clearer sense of social solidarity across generations rather than competition between them and to greater generosity in benefits that support child rearing. This view of child rearing as a contribution in kind to social security, a tax equivalent that should be recognized and compensated, is so different from most American discussions on social security and intergenerational relations that it needs some elaboration.

Children as Contributions in Kind

In all societies, economically active adults perform the labor that supports those who are not expected to work because of age, sickness, or disability. They also bear and rear children who will support them when they are no longer able to work. Protection against loss of income and poverty in old age, therefore, depends on a contract involving three generations. Where this intergenerational social security arrangement is informal and based on the family, the importance of children to their own parents' security is obvious. Grandparents are supported by their adult children, who also rear children who will in turn support their parents in their old age.

In societies with informal social security arrangements, having children and instilling in them a strong sense of filial obligation is the key to a person's security in old age. In the United States the 1910 census showed that for many adults, especially men, the informal insurance of children was what stood between them and the poorhouse in old age (Katz 1986). A formal social security system collectivizes this relation, while substituting a special tax, or contribution, system for reliance on filial piety. It remains true for the society that if a secure old age is to be ensured to its citizens, the society must rear children who will eventually work to support their elders.

In this formalization of social security, however, the direct link between rearing children as a young adult and economic security in old age is broken. It is only necessary that others rear children. Social Security, nevertheless, rests on two columns—the tax contributions that support current beneficiaries and the rearing of children who will constitute the next generation of workers and taxpayers. As Wattenberg (1987, 67) puts it, "Typically, we don't put money into the Social Security program for our own pensions. We put in babies."

The costs of child rearing are borne primarily by parents, but the benefits of social insurance reward occupational success, not parenting. By relating public pensions to prior earnings, social security systems typically penalize parents, especially mothers, rather than compensate them. They tax earnings without regard to family size and pay reduced benefits to people whose child-rearing activities have resulted in smaller lifetime earnings.

Some nations have long recognized the contribution in kind made by parents on behalf of their generation and have compensated them more or less directly for it through maternity benefits, paid parental leaves with job protection, housing subsidies, family allowances, and many other measures (Adams 1990). The Austrian legislature, for example, as long ago as 1950 recognized that "the burden of family maintenance . . . must be equalized between those who carry the burden in the interests of society as a whole and those who do not have to carry such burdens but consciously or unconsciously derive benefit from the fact that others do so for them" (Münz and Wintersberger 1984, 3).

In the 1970s and 1980s, in the face of concern about the present and future ratio of social security beneficiaries to contributors, there was in several countries a more explicit recognition of the dependence of retirement benefits on the contribution in kind made by those who rear children (see, for example, Andre and Burchardt 1980). Not only were child or family allowances (universal benefits for all families with children) increased in value in countries with aging populations, but parents were given credit within the social security system for child rearing as if it were equivalent to a period of covered employment—

one year per child, for example. Or the number of years of covered employment required to qualify for benefits was reduced, greatly increasing the numbers of women who received pensions (see Adams 1990 for details). One German plan proposed charging parents progressively lower social security taxes for life in proportion to the number of children they reared (Müller and Burkhardt 1983).

If there is a demographic imperative through which population aging shapes social policy, therefore, there is good reason to see it as impelling more rather than less public support for children and their parents (Ozawa 1986a, 1986b).

Age, Class, and Inequality

Analysis of spending patterns and demographic change in advanced capitalist democracies, however, shows that there is no clear pattern associating an aging population with either more or less spending for children. In some countries, like the United States and Japan, more elders and fewer children produce low spending for children; in others, like Sweden, Austria, and the Netherlands, similar demographic trends are associated with increasingly generous public transfers for children. Only when an aging population is combined with political or institutional factors does a clear pattern emerge that explains why the United States differs significantly from many European countries in its policy response to children and elders.

A recent study examined the effects of demographic change and political structure on family allowance expenditures between 1959 and 1986 in eighteen industrial democracies with mature welfare states (Pampel and Adams 1992). This time span includes both a period of expansion in these economies and their levels of social spending and a period of economic crisis and retrenchment following the oil shocks of the 1970s. Family allowances are not the only means of providing public support to offset the costs of child rearing, any more than old-age insurance is the only mechanism for supporting elders. They are, however, a good measure of the depth and effectiveness of political support for children and families. Other measures, like tax allowances, make little difference to national rankings or patterns (Pampel and Adams 1992; Pampel 1994). Family allowances are only a small part of family income, especially for the affluent, but they make an important contribution to preventing poverty for many families.

The study finds that an age structure with a high proportion of elderly people does not necessarily or typically reduce spending for children. It has greater influence on family allowance spending in democratic corporatist nations—that is, those like Austria and the Netherlands with nationally organized and centralized labor unions that negotiate with central government and employers' organizations—but the effect is to increase family allowance spending. In corporatist nations, an aging population increases spending for children.

Democratic corporatism is closely linked to leftist government, indicated by the degree to which social-democratic or labor parties with a strong working-class electoral base participate in national governments. The effect of the percentage of the aged in the population on family allowance spending in a country with no leftist government, like the United States or Japan, is near zero, whereas the effect for a nation with near-continuous thirty-year leftist government, like Sweden or Norway, is strongly positive.

In short, a high percentage of aged persons and a corporatist-leftist government interact to raise family allowance spending. These findings are consistent with a view that, in particular institutional conditions, programs for children are associated with programs for older citizens and do not compete against them. The United States, where issues of intergenerational equity have generated much debate, is atypical. For many advanced industrial democracies, an older age structure promotes, along with higher pension spending, a concern with the demographic implications for future pension financing and, thereby, support for child and family programs. Population aging in those countries highlights the importance of sharing the costs of rearing children who will contribute to the maintenance of their elders in the future.

Pampel (1994) extends this analysis by including public pensions along with family allowances. He developed a measure of age inequality, or bias, in public spending by determining the normative relationship between the two types of spending for the years and countries studied and then examining each country's distance from the norm. This approach avoids assuming either that there is an absolute, proper level of spending for each age group or that spending for one is causally related to spending for the other. The results show that "a large aged population reduces age inequality in favor of the elderly in the presence of (1) class-based corporatism and (2) strong leftist parties, whereas a large aged population increases age inequality in the absence of these two factors" (153).

The Politics of Generational Equity

All this shows that an increasing proportion of elderly people does not in itself increase or decrease spending for children, nor does it increase or decrease the relative share of spending going to older adults compared with children. High spending for the older population does not by itself produce intergenerational conflict. The impact of demographic change on public spending is shaped by political and institutional factors. What distinguishes the United States from other countries with as low or lower fertility and an age structure that is as old or older appears to be the political context—the way in which group interests are identified and organized to influence policy.

The view that the elderly use their numbers and political clout to compete with the young for social spending assumes a political environment of competing interest groups, based on age, gender, region, race, industry, class, and other characteristics. Interests organize themselves into an indefinite number of such groups that compete to influence policy relevant to narrowly defined goals. As Pampel (1994, 158) puts it, "Bargaining thus promotes concerns with particular programs in which specialized groups have direct interests, such as pensions for the aged or unemployment benefits for workers. The absence of (1) powerful class-based parties with ideologically coherent programs and (2) a correspondingly strong labor movement in pluralist nations both reinforces and is reinforced by these particularistic tendencies."

In contrast, where working classes have organized strong labor movements and political parties, they have not only succeeded in promoting and defending welfare states that provide extensive social protection for people in their roles as workers, parents, children, and elders but have also tended to generate bargaining processes that reinforce and are reinforced by universalist and solidaristic bonds across age groups. There is likely to be more concern with inequality within age cohorts and across the lifespan than between groups defined by age at a particular point in time and without regard to class. A picture begins to emerge of a U.S. political context characterized by interest group pluralism with a weak and fragmented labor movement and no labor party, in contrast to some European countries with strong, centralized labor movements, long periods of leftist government, and class-based corporatist bargaining structures. This picture, however, requires some further modification.

The absence of a socialist or labor party in the United States backed by a strong labor movement does not so much negate the importance of class in shaping U.S. social policy as it obscures it. Social Security represented a shift of part of the national wage bill from the market to the democratic political process. By sharing the support for elders among workers of all ages with or without dependent elderly parents and socializing the risks of income loss due to old age, disability, or death of a worker, Social Security reduced the economic insecurity of all wage-earning families. It both strengthened the security, and hence the bargaining position, of labor and achieved for capital a rationalization via the state of the costs of reproducing labor power from generation to generation (Adams 1985). It made retirement possible and so increased the efficiency of the labor force. And it responded to a political crisis of confidence and legitimacy in the midst of the Great Depression and gave workers a long-term stake in the system. It was an expression, not of an intergenerational struggle won by elders, but of an ongoing struggle and negotiation between capital and labor (Myles 1986).

Seen in this light, it becomes clear why those economists, politicians, and business leaders who raise the issue of generational equity want to "cut the graybeards a smaller slice of the pie" (Becker 1994, 20). It is not because they want to increase spending for children and families. Rather, they hope to extend the attack on public spending for families to the much more popular and better defended entitlement programs for elderly people. Rather than spreading the increased economic well-being achieved by older Americans through Social Security to the young, they want to erode elders' benefits as well. Their program is part of a larger effort to privatize the welfare state, involving less social protection for workers and their families and greater dependence on wages, private savings, and markets. The aim is reversion to a poor law type, residual social policy (Quadagno 1990).

In short, the critique of Social Security on grounds of generational equity can be understood as part of a (recently one-sided) class war that has succeeded in widening the gap between rich and poor and in increasing economic insecurity (Adams and Freeman 1982; Piven and Cloward 1982). It is a measure of the strength of capital and its two parties in the United States that such a class offensive can be disguised as a conflict between generations. It is also a mark of the strength and success of the Social Security system that such an ideological smoke-screen should be necessary.

Conclusion

Efforts in the United States to promote a politics of generational equity are best understood as part of a larger class struggle over the welfare state, an important aspect of which is the attempt to define the conflict in terms of age rather than class. That this age-based politics has some resonance in the United States (and little if any in other countries) is itself an expression of a particular combination of demographic and political circumstances and is not the inevitable outcome of population aging.

Leftist government and a policy making structure that enables a strong and centralized labor movement to bargain at the national level not only reduce age inequality (while rightist rule and a fragmented interest group pluralism increase it) but also make for generous welfare states in general, with less poverty for children and elders. Those on the political right who attack Social Security and other programs for the older population are themselves in this sense part of the problem they decry. They support political parties, structures, and class interests that generate inequality between generations as well as between classes. Americans who wish to improve the position of children and to decrease spending bias in favor of older adults would do better to devote their energies to building a labor party and a strong labor movement.

[handwritten marginalia: all europe except switzerland]

There is good reason to acknowledge the link between old and young in relation to social security, though that relation is not grasped by the rhetoric of generational equity and competing interest groups. Measures that recognize the contribution in kind to society in general, and social security in particular, that child rearing involves, would build on rather than undermine the Social Security system, which has been so successful in reducing poverty among the older population. Such measures could include a universal family allowance program, reduced Social Security taxes, and increased benefits according to number of children reared, maternity benefits, and paid parental leaves. Programs of this sort can be designed to help equalize the burden of child rearing between parents and nonparents, and between men and women, while protecting maternal and infant health and improving the short- and long-term economic security and career prospects of women (Stoiber 1989; Adams 1990).

As universal benefits, such measures would not penalize work or stigmatize recipients, but they would disproportionately raise the incomes of low-income families with children. They would compensate those who contribute to Social Security not only through their covered employment but also through child rearing and who presently are penalized first by reduced lifetime earnings and again in retirement by lower earnings-related Social Security benefits. As a result, this approach would provide an important step toward the elimination of poverty among both children and women, including older women. It would further social solidarity between generations and improve the economic security of families throughout the life cycle.

References

Adams, P. 1985. Social Policy and the Working Class. *Social Service Review* 59:387–402.

———. 1990. Children as Contributions in Kind: Social Security and Family Policy. *Social Work* 35:492–98.

Adams, P., and G. Freeman. 1982. Social Services under Reagan and Thatcher. In N. Fainstein and S. Fainstein, eds., *Urban Policy under Capitalism.* Beverly Hills, Calif.: Sage.

Andre, A., and K. Burchardt. 1980. *Employment and Social Security in the Federal Republic of Germany.* St. Augustin: Asgar-Verlag Hippe for the Federal Ministry of Labor and Social Order.

Becker, G. 1994. Cut the Graybeards a Smaller Slice of the Pie. *Business Week,* Mar. 28.

Heclo, H. 1988. Generational Politics. In J. Palmer, T. Smeeding, and B. Torrey, eds., *The Vulnerable.* Washington, D.C.: Urban Institute.

Katz, M. 1986. *In the Shadow of the Poorhouse: A Social History of Welfare in America.* New York: Basic Books.

Koretz, G. 1995. Pitting Grandpa against Junior? *Business Week,* Apr. 3.

Müller, J., and W. Burkhardt. 1983. Die 3-Generationen-Solidarität in der Rentenversicherung als System-Notwendigkeit und ihre Konsequenzen [Three-Generation Solidarity in Pension Insurance as a Systemic Necessity and Its Consequences]. *Sozialer Fortschritt* 32:73–77.

Mhnz, R., and H. Wintersberger. 1984. The Austrian Welfare State: Social Policy and Income Maintenance Programmes between 1970 and 1984. *International Social Security Review* 37:303.

Myles, J. 1986. Citizenship at the Crossroads: The Future of Old Age Security. In D. Van Tassel and P. Stearns, eds., *Old Age in a Bureaucratic Society.* Westwood, Conn.: Greenwood.

Ozawa, M. 1986a. The Nation's Children: Key to a Secure Retirement. *New England Journal of Human Services* 6:12–19.

———. 1986b. Non-Whites and the Demographic Imperative in Social Welfare. *Social Work* 31:440–46.

Pampel, F. 1994. Population Aging, Class Context, and Age Inequality in Public Spending. *American Journal of Sociology* 100:153–95.

Pampel, F., and P. Adams. 1992. The Effects of Demographic Change and Political Structure on Family Allowance Expenditures. *Social Service Review* 66:524–46.

Piven, F., and R. Cloward. 1982. *The New Class War.* New York: Pantheon.

Preston, S. 1984. Children and the Elderly: Divergent Paths for America's Dependents. *Demography* 21:435–57.

Quadagno, J. 1990. Generational Equity and the Politics of the Welfare State. *International Journal of Health Services* 20:631–49.

Stoiber, S. 1989. *Parental Leave and "Woman's Place": The Implications and Impact of Three European Approaches to Family Leave Policy.* Washington, D.C.: Women's Research and Education Institute.

Wattenberg, B. 1987. *The Birth Dearth.* New York: Pharos.

PART III

POLICY ARENAS AND THE PLACE OF AGE

9

Social Security
Marketing Radical Reform

ERIC R. KINGSON and JILL QUADAGNO

Entitlement fever is hitting the nation, creating new opportunities for those seeking to radically alter the structure and terms of eligibility for Social Security. From the Concord Coalition's call to means-test Social Security, to the declaration of the 1995 Bipartisan Commission on Entitlement and Tax Reform that current federal commitments—largely to elderly people—unfairly burden the nation's children, to the furor over the balanced budget amendment, to the strenuous efforts of free marketers to privatize Social Security, efforts abound to legitimize radical change.

Although Social Security's projected financing problems are many years off, the Social Security rhetoric is already escalating to a feverish pitch. Testifying before the Bipartisan Commission, a self-appointed representative of "generation X" gleefully reports that more American adults under age thirty-five believe in UFOs than in the future of Social Security (Lukefahr 1994). The *Boston Globe* argues that Social Security is an immense Ponzi scheme that is slowly bankrupting young Americans to enrich their elders (Jacoby 1994). The cover of *Time* advertises "The Case for Killing Social Security," a feature article that says "the numbers don't add up—and the politicians won't own up" (Church and Lacayo 1995, 24). And advocates of privatization promise a hundred million millionaires, a secure old age, and a thriving economy for all if workers' payroll tax contributions could be converted to private savings accounts (see Beard 1996).

To date, there has been much hyperbole but little action. The Bipartisan Commission failed to agree on any proposals. Speaker of the House Newt Gingrich quickly professed that Social Security reform would remain off the table for at least six years, lest this potentially explosive issue derail the Contract with America. The balanced budget amendment stumbled in the Senate amid growing public fears that it would force large cuts in Social Security.

Even so, rhetoric matters, because how the problem is defined establishes the parameters for possible solutions. The financing problems of Social Security provide an important window of opportunity for those seeking to advance an agenda of lower taxes and smaller government. What is occurring now is the contentious process of setting an agenda to decide the future of the nation's most successful social policy—Social Security, the Old Age, Survivors, and Disability Insurance (OASDI) program. Proposals previously associated with the far right (most notably, partial privatization and means testing of Social Security) are now emerging as options requiring serious consideration. Indeed, the 1996 Advisory Council on Social Security seriously discussed—without reaching consensus—two plans that would redirect some portion of Social Security payroll tax contributions into private accounts. In this new political environment, other changes that, while less extreme, are still drastic (for example, raising the normal retirement age to seventy) have come to look like moderate alternatives. The potential consequences of such changes—for women, minorities, and poor people, and for the future of the middle class—are receiving little attention, a fact that should be of great concern.

Here, we first review the existing Social Security financing problem and then examine the perception of Social Security as a program in crisis, including the marketing of the program as a burden to young people. Next, we examine selected proposals for cutting Social Security that arise from a definition of the program as unfair and unsustainable. We conclude by discussing real solutions for restoring the long-range solvency of the Social Security trust fund, including the maintenance of benefits plan (advanced by six of the thirteen members of the 1996 Advisory Council on Social Security) that seeks to address the financing problem while maintaining the basic promises and structure of OASDI.

The Social Security Financing Problem

No doubt about it, there is a Social Security financing problem. Without any changes in current law, Social Security is projected to meet its obligations for the next thirty-three years. But under intermediate-cost assumptions, the Social Security trustees' report projects a shortfall of 2.19 percent of the payroll over the seventy-five-year period—1996 to 2070—over which long-range estimates are made. This represents a roughly 14 percent shortfall. Since the deficit years fall in the middle and at the end of the estimating period, the largest shortfalls in the out years (i.e., after 2035) are substantially greater than suggested by the overall 2.19 percent-of-payroll estimate (4.86% of the payroll from 2046 to 2070; see U.S. Federal Old-Age and Survivors 1996).

However, while the projected financing shortfall must be addressed, it constitutes a warning, not a crisis. Tax returns (payroll tax receipts and receipts from taxation of benefits) will exceed outlays until 2012. Total income, including interest earnings, is expected to exceed expenditures through 2018 (by $60 billion in 1995 alone) and the combined OASDI trust fund is projected to meet all its commitments through 2028, with sufficient revenues to meet 76 percent of all benefits promised thereafter (ibid.). Of course, the projected shortfall may be larger or smaller, depending on economic and demographic changes.

A Program in Crisis?

The facts surrounding Social Security financing are not in dispute. The meaning attributed to the projected financing problem, however, is the source of lively debate. A new set of political circumstances has led to the definition of Social Security—both implicitly and explicitly—as a major problem, part of an "entitlement crisis" (Quadagno 1995, 1996). This view is incubated by budget politics and anxiety over the future and thrives in the presence of stereotypes of "greedy geezers," distortions about the value of Social Security, and a simplistic view of entitlements as a single entity. It is supported by a flawed but seemingly objective analysis of the size and implications of the federal deficit.

Crafting a Message of Fear

For some critics of Social Security, the strategy of tying Social Security to the rhetoric of an "entitlement crisis" is a carefully conceived and executed strategy to shrink the federal government and advance the idea that radical reforms are needed in Social Security and other social programs. Frank Luntz (1995), a pollster who worked on the Contract with America, advised in a memo to the new Republican congressional majority that the budget debate should be cast "in terms of 'the American dream' and 'our children's future.'" To survive and prosper as a movement, Luntz said, Republicans must frame questions in moral terms, not in the heartless language of "budgeteers." And, he told them, they must turn "the issue of 'fairness' against the Democrats," asking such questions as, "Is it 'fair' for Medicare recipients to have an even greater choice of doctors and facilities than the average taxpayers who are funding the system?" Similarly, according to the final report of the U.S. Bipartisan Commission on Entitlement and Tax Reform (1995, ii), "Left unchecked, the Federal government's long-term spending commitments on entitlement programs . . . will lead to excessively high deficit and debt levels, unfairly burdening America's children and stifling standards of living for this and future generations of Americans."

Although Social Security, the "third rail of American politics," is often considered "too hot to touch," its being framed as an out-of-control entitlement that benefits the "wrong people" (the poor, the rich, or the middle class, depending on the critic's argument) may provide a back door to a radical destructuring of the program. Journalists, politicians, and budget advocates who approach the issue in this manner consistently highlight the program's various problems (financing, declining rates of return as the system matures, women's equity and adequacy concerns, declining public confidence) while ignoring its overall success. This image of the program as a drain on hard-working Americans and the young (as if they and their families do not face risks associated with disability, retirement, or death) is bolstered by analyses purporting to show that the growth of Social Security is part of a "unitary entitlement problem" that, left unchecked, will bankrupt the future. Thus the interim report of the U.S. Bipartisan Commission on Entitlement and Tax Reform contends that "unless appropriate policy changes are made in the interim, projected outlays for entitlements and interest on the national debt will consume all tax revenues collected by the federal government" (1994, 6). Entitlements do indeed seem out of control.

Separate Programs, Separate Problems

Lumping all entitlements together as one large problem creates a false sense of crisis and places obstacles in the path of realistic reform of Social Security financing. There are many entitlement programs, each serving important social purposes and each in need of a thoughtful, ongoing review. The two major programs—Social Security and Medicare, which together account for 60 percent of entitlement spending—are both in need of reform, but for different reasons and in different ways. In fact, the entitlement "crisis" looks quite different when entitlements are separated according to specific programs. Social Security's outlay as a share of the gross domestic product (GDP) is forecast as growing from only 4.7 percent in 1996 to 6.6 percent by 2030. Even modest reductions in benefit levels would reduce that share. A 1.6 percent growth in share of the GDP is not a terribly heavy price to pay for the retirement security of the baby boom cohort, whose education, employment, and housing needs we have been able to meet thus far without sacrificing economic security. What's more, many of our economic competitors devote a considerably higher proportion of their GDP to public pensions without raising the alarm that pervades Washington today. The percentage of the GDP spent on pensions ranges from 15.03 in Austria to 11.87 in Sweden to 4.97 in Japan, compared to the 4.8 percent figure for the United States (Organization for Economic Cooperation and Development 1994).

The rest of the so-called entitlement problem is caused by other programs, mostly Medicare and Medicaid, and by interest on the debt. Projected long-term federal deficits are driven primarily by rapidly increasing health care costs and only secondarily by anticipated increases in Social Security expenditures. Medicare and Medicaid costs have been growing rapidly, and the Medicare Hospital Insurance trust fund is projected to be depleted in 2001. Congress is currently considering measures to reduce health care inflation and bring the spiraling costs of Medicare and Medicaid under control. If any of these measures succeeds, the "crisis" lessens.

Notwithstanding the differing functions of the various entitlement programs and the differing challenges they face, the advocates of radical change prefer to talk about Social Security's financing problems as if Social Security, Medicare, Medicaid, and the many other entitlement programs were a single entity—all part of one big entitlement crisis. Proposals advanced by the Concord Coalition and by individual members of the Bipartisan Commission provide case examples of the solutions that emerge from this framework.

Social Security Reforms within the Framework of an "Entitlement Crisis"

Deficit politics are lending new legitimacy to proposals to reform Social Security by means testing, privatization, and greatly scaling back benefits. While these proposals are often portrayed as a way to reduce long-run federal deficits, what gets lost are the human consequences of such proposals as well as their long-term effects on the future of the program. What follows is a look at some of these proposals, especially their impact on the Social Security program and on low-income workers, minorities, and women, groups that depend far more heavily on Social Security than do other recipient populations.

A Social Security Means Test

As the central feature of its deficit-cutting strategy, the Concord Coalition (1993) advances Peter Peterson's proposal of a comprehensive means test (also knows as the affluence test) of Social Security and many other entitlements. The coalition is proposing to reduce Social Security and other benefit payments for higher-income beneficiaries. In contrast to most means-tested programs, which rely on welfare bureaucracies to determine who is poor enough to receive social benefits, the new approach would use a means test applied through the tax system to reduce benefits for the more affluent beneficiaries of Social Security and a variety of other federal social insurance and public assistance programs (ibid.). Income from Social Security, unemployment insurance, welfare programs, selected veterans' benefits, farm payments, and the insurance value of Medicare would be subject to a graduated reduction—ranging from 10 to 85 percent—when income from all sources exceeds $40,000. Households with $55,000, $95,000, and $120,000 in income would lose 15, 55, and 85 percent of their benefits, respectively. In no case would the reduction exceed 85 percent (see Concord Coalition 1993; Peterson 1995). Peterson (58) suggests that an "affluence test" will strengthen Social Security while meeting the fairness challenge of achieving "large fiscal savings without hurting low-income Americans." But would it?

Indeed, this approach goes a long way toward answering two criticisms of means-tested programs—that they are administratively complex and that they stigmatize beneficiaries (Kingson and Schulz 1997). But it does not address the main criticisms—that means testing would initiate a process that is likely to pull apart America's most successful social policy and, in the long run, to be particularly harmful to low- and moderate-income households (Kingson 1994; Kingson and Schulz 1997). Failure to provide some reasonable return to higher-income people who contribute to Social Security over their entire work lives would inevitably lead to demands by these people to withdraw from the program. Social Security is already criticized by some higher-income workers as not giving them their "money's worth"; means testing would further fuel their discontent. Without the political support and participation of affluent people, there would be no way to sustain the progressivity of the program's benefit formula, which returns roughly twice as much to low-income people as to high-income people while simultaneously extending broad protection to the middle class (Ball and Aaron 1993).

Moreover, means testing of Social Security, Medicare, and other social insurance entitlements would discourage savings (Ball 1994; Bernstein 1990; Myers 1994; Steuerle 1994; Walker 1994) and would introduce a new level of uncertainty into retirement income planning. By reducing Social Security, Medicare, and other social insurance benefits of savers by as much as 85 percent, the government would be sending a message that it values consumption over retirement savings. Moreover, Quadagno (1996, 398) notes that by providing a different set of incentives for higher-income persons, means-testing and privatization efforts threaten to "undermine the moral framework that has sustained public support for Social Security by fracturing solidarity along lines of class and of generations."

Changes in Benefits and Eligibility Age

Senator J. Robert Kerrey (D-Nebraska) and former Senator John Danforth (R-Missouri) propose a solution to the "entitlement crisis" that includes changing the Social Security benefit formula and raising the age of eligibility for benefits. The combined impact of their proposals would be a 43 percent cut in Social Security benefits. The burden of these cuts would be particularly damaging to people in low-income households. The most problematic benefit cut involves a technical change in the benefit formula that, beginning in 1998, would index the Social Security "bend points" for inflation instead of for average wage growth. Under current law, two calculations are used to determine the amount of a worker's initial benefits.

First, the worker's average indexed monthly earnings (AIME) figure is calculated based on the worker's earnings record (of wages that were subject to the payroll tax). This calculation involves adjusting all covered wages for changes in average wages that have occurred since the year in which the wages were earned (indexed to age sixty). These amounts are then averaged together with any wages for age sixty and after to produce the AIME. This procedure helps ensure that benefits based on earnings keep pace with real wage growth, not just with inflation.

Second, the primary insurance amount (PIA) is calculated. The PIA is the basic monthly benefit, equivalent to the monthly benefit received by a worker retiring at normal retirement age. In 1996, the PIA benefit formula replaces 90 percent of the first $437 of AIME, 32 percent of the next $2,198 of AIME, and 15 percent of AIME in excess of $2,635.

The dollar amounts at which the percentage rates in this formula change are called "bend points." These bend points are also wage indexed—increased annually by the growth in average wages. The percentage rates in the PIA formula do not change. The wage indexing of the bend points helps guarantee that, over time, Social Security benefits reflect changes in average wages and replace a fairly constant proportion of preretirement earnings for workers at comparable wage levels.

Under the Kerrey-Danforth proposal, as real wages rise over time, all new beneficiaries would get pushed into a higher bend point bracket, and thus replacement rates (and benefit amounts) would eventually decline, with the younger cohorts experiencing much greater reductions. This change would undermine protections extended to poor people, because more of their income would be replaced at 32 percent and less at 90 percent. The effect would be greatest on beneficiaries who receive a proportionately larger share of their incomes from Social Security—namely, poor people, aged widows of the future, and low-wage workers. Moreover, instead of stabilizing Social Security financing, tying bend points to changes in the consumer price index instead of changes in average wages would increase financing pressures during periods of high inflation and low growth. It would result in larger benefit increases during periods of low wage growth and high inflation.

The Kerrey-Danforth Social Security proposal also includes a plan to gradually raise the normal retirement age to seventy. Currently, the age of eligibility for full retirement benefits is sixty-five. Beginning in the next century, it will gradually increase to age sixty-seven over a twenty-seven-year period. When fully implemented, early retirement benefits will be reduced, with benefits declining at age sixty-two from 80 percent of a full benefit to 70 percent, for example.

In many respects, it makes sense to raise the retirement age. People are living longer. Many have better health than in the past and are capable of working longer. The main effect of this option, however, would not be to delay retirement and keep older people in the labor force (Sammartino 1987; Leonesio 1993): simulations of the effect of the increase in the normal retirement age to sixty-seven suggest that the average age of receipt of benefits will increase by only two to three months (Gustman and Steinmeier 1985). Rather, the primary effect would be to produce long-run savings for Social Security by reducing early retirement benefits and the value of benefits at normal retirement age. Increases in the normal age of retirement will also result in benefit reductions for aged spouses and aged widows and widowers. Reductions in benefits for the latter two groups are especially problematic, given their economic insecurity.

An increase of the retirement age to seventy would mean a 40 percent cut in benefits for workers retiring at age sixty-two. The burden of the proposed change would fall most heavily on lower-income early retirees (see Sammartino 1987), most notably older workers in poor health, older workers who are functionally limited (but not totally disabled), minority older workers, unemployed older workers, and early retirees in downsizing industries. The combined impact of the benefit formula and retirement age changes would be a whopping 43 percent cut in Social Security benefits.

More recently, Senator Kerrey teamed up with former Senator Alan Simpson (R-Wyoming) to offer a revised version of the Kerrey-Danforth plan, termed the Personal Investment Plan Act of 1995. While still raising the retirement age to seventy and containing a substantial reduction in benefits via benefit formula changes, the revised plan includes very significant reductions in cost-of-living protections. By limiting full COLA (cost-of-living adjustment) protection to the portion of an individual's benefit that is equal to 30 percent of the median Social Security benefit (i.e., the individual's PIA), this proposal would especially impair the economic security of formerly middle-income women living to advanced old age. On average, the combined impact of the Kerrey-Simpson bill would be a 33 percent cut in benefits.

Privatization

Big benefit cuts are needed, according to the Kerrey-Danforth approach, to fund a giant step in the direction of privatizing Social Security—a 1.5 percent payroll tax decrease (2% under Kerrey-Simpson) for everyone under age fifty-five, along with a requirement that this money be placed in a personal savings (IRA-like) account. Contributions to the individual personal account would not be deductible, and earnings on the account would be taxed on withdrawal. Withdrawal would be allowed only on disability or retirement.

Because the Social Security trust fund will become insolvent by 2030, the logical solution to restoring solvency might be to raise payroll taxes. But the Kerrey-Danforth option would *cut* payroll taxes. The rationale for cutting payroll taxes is based on the argument that such a cut would promote savings and personal responsibility. Right now, there is little evidence that privatization of benefits would have any effect on national savings, since it would merely shift funds from public to private accounts. Also, there is no evidence that this reduction in payroll taxes would provide an adequate substitute for Social Security benefits. Rather, experience suggests that people would be likely to withdraw these funds and use them as family needs arose, unless the system were highly regulated. The real impact would simply be to jeopardize the trust funds and reduce income security in old age.

Even so, proposals for privatization are proliferating. Two plans emerging out of the 1996 Advisory Council on Social Security—the individual account (IA), supported by two (of thirteen) members, and the personal security account (PSA), supported by five members—would also radically depart from the sixty-year tradition of gradual Social Security reform. Both would introduce mandatory private savings through individual accounts.

The IA plan would raise the normal retirement age and scale back replacement rates for higher-income workers (Gramlich forthcoming). The PSA plan would dramatically alter Social Security by phasing in a two-tier system—a universal flat benefit equal to two-thirds of the poverty line and individual accounts whose value would reflect the outcome of the earnings and investment decisions of workers (see Schieber, this volume). Both plans, especially the PSA, address the thorny transition problems posed by privatization proposals by reducing benefit commitments under the basic OASDI program while also increasing revenues. The IA plan would mandate a 1.6 percent payroll charge. The PSA plan contains a seventy-five-year transition payroll tax of 1.5 percent, with additional borrowing from general revenues during the first third of the twenty-first century. Besides addressing the financing problem, proponents of these options see them as promoting the savings habit and assuring younger workers that their Social Security investments will come to fruition. Their opponents see these plans as reducing—dramatically so for the PSA plan—benefits payable under the Social Security program, shifting additional risks associated with economic fluctuations onto individuals, and compromising the antipoverty role of Social Security. Some see these plans as, by explicitly separating out the individual equity and adequacy components of OASDI, potentially undermining political support for the program, especially its poverty reduction features (see Ball 1995; Gramlich forthcoming; Quinn and Mitchell 1996).

Relatively little thought has been given to what the private retirement accounts would look like, how they would be managed, and what fees might be charged by private investors to manage the accounts. These issues have implications both for the income security of retirees and for the economy. Will there be any governmental supervision of how workers invest these funds? Or will workers be able to simply take the extra dollars and invest them as they please? Some proposals imply that the only penalty on workers for withdrawing funds from these accounts is that they will be taxed. If early withdrawals are allowed, experience suggests that workers may take the money out to pay off other debts, due to life events like illness or divorce, and pay the tax penalty. If withdrawals are not allowed, what gigantic government agency will be put in place to monitor the private savings accounts of millions of individuals? To keep the Social Security trust fund solvent, the payroll tax cut must be accompanied by the benefit cuts discussed above. The implicit assumption is that returns from private investments will make up the difference in retirement income. Perhaps some workers would do better, but others may lose all their money through poor investments or bad advice. Thus, retirement savings could decline further rather than increase.

Senator Alan Simpson and Representatives Alex McMillan and Porter Goss proposed an alternative privatization plan in the Bipartisan Commission's final report. Their plan would make opting out of payroll taxes voluntary. If opting out becomes voluntary, then one must consider the effect on the entire system. Currently, the taxes of higher-income workers subsidize the benefits of low-income workers.

One likely scenario is that high-income workers would opt out but low-income workers would remain. That is in fact what happened in Great Britain, because the setup costs of the optional plans made opting out too costly for low-income workers (Daykin 1994).

If high earners opt out, would there still be sufficient tax contributions to pay low-income retirees what they are promised? If opting out makes it impossible to pay promised benefits to low-income retirees, where would the money come from? General revenues? An increase in payroll taxes? If opting out isn't established as some form of a mandatory defined contribution plan, then the proposal could merely amount to a payroll tax decrease for those workers who opt out. Under a voluntary system, how would opting out be operationalized? Employers' bookkeeping would become much more complex. Firms would have some workers paying full payroll taxes and others paying reduced payroll taxes. Further, workers could choose to opt out at various points in time. Administration would also become more complex for the Social Security Administration. These costs need to be factored into the estimates of how this option would affect the federal budget and how it would affect firms.

Discussion of options like those reviewed above has yet to take place in a public forum. Some, such as retirement age increases, are perfectly reasonable to consider as part of a balanced package, but taken together, "solutions" such as those advanced in the Kerrey-Danforth and the Kerrey-Simpson packages do much more than is needed to restore the trust funds to actuarial balance. What these proposals and many other privatization proposals have in common is one more version of rolling back the federal government. Instead of returning programs to the states, however, they return income security in old age to the private sector, providing clear benefits to some (for example, investment portfolio managers), increased uncertainty for many, and clear losses to those with little protection beyond Social Security.

Options for Social Security Reform within the Existing Structure

The above critique is not intended to suggest that the projected financing problem should be ignored. Quite the contrary. While no immediate crisis exists, there is a need to advance policies—perhaps some combination of benefit reductions and tax increases—that will put the program back into actuarial balance. Changes affecting the income of future retirees should be put in place with sufficient lead time for workers to adjust their retirement expectations and savings behavior. Moreover, postponing action for many years would further undermine public confidence in the program and serve as an invitation to crisis mongering and sensational news reporting.

The Social Security trust fund can be restored to long-range solvency with relatively minor adjustments rather than a major restructuring of the program. Robert Ball (1995), former commissioner of Social Security, notes that "there are many ways of bringing Social Security into long-range balance within the principles of the program." What might a plan look like?

The Maintenance of Benefits Plan

Six of the thirteen members of the Advisory Council on Social Security support one such plan, the maintenance of benefits plan. This plan begins with four proposals essentially supported by almost all members of the council:

• Extending coverage to new state and local government employees (most are already covered).

• Reducing benefits by roughly 3 percent by computing average earnings of future beneficiaries based on thirty-eight years of earnings (instead of thirty-five).

• Taxing Social Security benefits in roughly the same manner as income from contributory, defined benefit plans.

• Adjusting the COLA to reflect the Bureau of Labor Statistics estimate that the consumer price index overadjusts for inflation by 0.21 percent.

Together, these changes would reduce the projected financing problem by about 1.06 percent of the taxable payroll—that is, they would address nearly half of the projected seventy-five-year average annual deficit of 2.17 percent of the taxable payroll. Additionally, the maintenance of benefits plan would:

• Direct (by 2020) all income generated from taxing OASDI into the combined OASDI trust fund. (A portion of these receipts is credited currently to the Medicare Hospital Insurance trust fund.)

• Schedule a 1.6 percent payroll tax increase (0.8% on employer and employee) near the middle of the twenty-first century.

• And, very importantly, gradually invest two-fifths of OASDI trust fund assets in broad, passively managed index funds (e.g., Wilshire 5000). (This change would indirectly increase rates of return to individuals while also eliminating 40 percent [+.90% of the taxable payroll] of the projected financing problem.)

Proponents of this plan note that it addresses financing problems (leaving a margin of safety) and improves the rate of return on Social Security contributions, while maintaining the basic promises and structure of OASDI.

These options would solve the problem. They are not the only options. And they should be subject to the same analysis of consequences as those discussed above. Computing benefits over thirty-eight years instead of thirty-five years would primarily represent a benefit cut for higher-income people, who begin work later in life than blue-collar workers do. The practice could disadvantage some women, however, who leave the labor force to care for children or elderly parents. Similarly, a 1.6 percent payroll tax increase is an increase in a regressive tax, and investing trust fund assets in the private sector would introduce new volatility in trust fund financing.

Other Reforms to Preserve Social Security

Even if one does not like the maintenance of benefits plan, it is important to recognize that many other reforms could address the financing problems of the program without dramatically altering the distribution of benefits and obligations or the structure of the program. Starting with the four common elements of the three Advisory Council plans (-1.09% of taxable payroll savings), here are some other incremental changes that are consistent with the existing Social Security program.

The widening of the income gap in the United States—the upper-income quintile's share having risen from 45.1 percent in 1983 to 48.3 percent ten years later—could be viewed as providing the rationale for adjusting the taxable maximum ceiling, set at $62,700 in 1996. Another proposal would restore and maintain the proportion of wages covered by the payroll tax—now at 88 percent and projected to drop to 85.5 percent in ten years—at the 90 percent level by 2000. This would address about 14 percent of the projected financing problem.

In a similar vein, one could argue that increased burden should be placed on firms offering disproportionately high salaries by subjecting 100 percent of the employer's payroll to FICA taxation. Doing so would be consistent with the view that the employer's contribution is part of a pool of funds that promotes the social goals of Social Security, including proportionately larger benefits for low- and moderate-income beneficiaries. Leaving the employee share capped would eliminate the need to increase benefits for future beneficiaries, as would be the case for proposals that would eliminate the maximum taxable ceiling from both employers and employees. If implemented in 1998, lifting the ceiling on the employer share would address about half of the projected problem.

In place of raising the maximum taxable ceiling, one could select from among the plethora of moderate reform alternatives—raising the retirement age to sixty-eight, reducing the percentage of the last bend point, or cutting the spouse benefit—and still restore actuarial balance. Others might treat some portion of fringe benefits as taxable for Social Security purposes or return to an entirely pay-as-you-go system (with a floating tax rate). The point is, as the plan illustrates, the financing problem can be addressed without privatizing, means-testing, or otherwise altering the basic structure of the program. And many benefit changes can be made without making wrenching cuts and without the destabilizing effects of switching to a consumer price index measure for bend points adjustments or greatly reducing cost-of-living protections.

Assuming modest growth (for example, 1.3 to 2 percent real growth) over the next thirty to sixty years, the United States should be able to respond to the strains in program financing that will accompany population aging without placing undue burden on future cohorts of workers. If the economy grows at rates that are greater than anticipated, then it will be easier to respond to financing challenges. If the growth is slower, further adjustments in Social Security will be needed. Perhaps the most realistic way of responding to the inevitable uncertainties that surround financial projections is to put in place one set of changes (for example, some combination of payroll tax increases and benefit reductions) around 2020, when, as currently expected, we will begin to draw down trust fund reserves. A second set of changes could be scheduled in 2035, structured in such a way as to capture greater savings in the out years when the gap between anticipated income and costs is expected to be largest. Having scheduled such adjustments, we should expect that we will return to Social Security financing many times before 2070 and make changes as future experience proves better or worse than currently anticipated.

Conclusion

The Social Security trustees have sounded a warning bell, not a fire alarm, as the program's opponents are fond of suggesting. Social Security can be brought into long-range actuarial balance without destroying a system that has reduced poverty and provided income security in old age, survivor's insurance to nearly every American, and protection against disability—all without ever missing a payment. Public discourse needs to move past the tendency to reduce discussions about Social Security to accounting exercises that focus only on program costs, overlooking the benefits this program provides and the real consequences to the well-being of individuals and families that various possible changes may have.

Social Security is an institution that has strengthened the nation's families and communities. In a very fundamental way, it is an expression of the moral commitment of our nation to serve as our brothers', sisters', fathers', mothers', and our own keepers. In the process of addressing long-term financing problems, we should lose sight of neither the economic implications of various policy options nor the moral dimensions of this program, which is one of the joining institutions of our society.

References

Ball, R. 1994. Testimony before the Bipartisan Commission on Entitlement and Tax Reform. July 15.

———. 1995. Letter to members of Bipartisan Commission on Entitlement and Tax Reform. Jan. 9.

Ball, R., and H. Aaron. 1993. The Myth of Means Testing. *Washington Post,* Nov. 14.

Beard, S. 1996. *Restoring Hope in America: The Social Security Solution.* San Francisco: Institute for Contemporary Studies.

Bernstein, M. 1990. Social Security: Continued Entitlement or New Means Test? An Issue of Program Stability. *Research Dialogues* 26:1B8.

Church, G., and R. Lacayo. 1995. Social Security: The Numbers Don't Add Up—and the Politicians Won't Own Up. *Time,* Mar. 20.

Concord Coalition. 1993. *The Zero Deficit Plan.* Washington, D.C.

Daykin, C. 1994. Occupational Pension Provision in the United Kingdom. Paper presented at the 1994 Pension Research Council Symposium, "Security Employer-Based Pensions: An International Perspective," Wharton School, University of Pennsylvania, May 5–6.

Gramlich, N. Forthcoming. Different Approaches for Dealing with Social Security. *Journal of Economic Perspectives.*

Gustman, A., and T. Steinmeier. 1985. The 1983 Social Security Reforms and Labor Supply Adjustments of Older Individuals in the Long Run. *Journal of Labor Economics* 3:237B53.

Jacoby, J. 1994. The Social Security Scam. *Boston Globe,* Dec. 20.

Kingson, E. 1994. Testing the Boundaries of Universality: What's Mean? What's Not? *Gerontologist* 34:735B39.

Kingson, E., and J. Schulz. 1997. Should Social Security Be Means-Tested? In J. Schulz and E. Kingson, eds., *Social Security in the Twenty-First Century.* New York: Oxford University Press.

Leonesio, M. 1993. Social Security and Older Workers. *Social Security Bulletin* 56:47B58.

Lukefahr, R. 1994. Testimony before the Bipartisan Commission on Entitlement and Tax Reform. Sept. 23.

Luntz, F. 1995. Memorandum to the Republican Conference (Jan. 9) as reproduced in the *New York Times,* Feb. 5.

Myers, R. 1994. Testimony before the Bipartisan Commission on Entitlement and Tax Reform. July 15.

Organization for Economic Cooperation and Development. 1994. *New Orientations for Social Policy.* Paris.

Peterson, P. 1995. Reform Proposal of Commissioner Peter G. Peterson. In Bipartisan Commission on Entitlement and Tax Reform, *Final Report to the President,* Washington, D.C.

Quadagno, J. 1995. The Myth of the Entitlement Crisis. Paper presented at the American Sociological Association's Congressional Briefing, March 6, Washington, D.C.

———. 1996. Social Security and the Myth of the Entitlement Crisis. *Gerontologist* 36:391–99.

Quinn, J., and O. Mitchell. 1996. Social Security on the Table. *American Prospect* (May–June): 76–81.

Sammartino, F. 1987. The Effect of Health on Retirement. *Social Security Bulletin* 50:41.

Steuerle, C. 1994. Testimony before the Bipartisan Commission on Entitlement and Tax Reform. July 15.

U.S. Bipartisan Commission on Entitlement and Tax Reform. 1994. *Interim Report to the President.* Washington, D.C.

———. 1995. *Final Report to the President.* Washington, D.C.

U.S. Federal Old-Age and Survivors Insurance and Disability Insurance Trust Funds, Board of Trustees. 1995. *Annual Report of the Federal Old-Age and Survivors Insurance and Disability Insurance Trust Funds.* Washington, D.C.: Government Printing Office.

———. 1996. *Annual Report of the Federal Old-Age and Survivors Insurance and Disability Insurance Trust Funds.* Washington, D.C.: Government Printing Office.

U.S. Social Security Administration. 1995. Social Security Trustees Release Annual Report. Press release, Apr. 3.

Walker, D. 1994. Testimony before the Bipartisan Commission on Entitlement and Tax Reform, July 15. Washington, D.C.

10

A New Vision for Social Security
*Personal Security Accounts as an Element
of Social Security Reform*

SYLVESTER J. SCHIEBER

A proposal that I and a group of other members of the 1996 Social
Security Advisory Council put forth would significantly change the
current structure of Social Security. Each worker would contribute a
portion of his or her payroll taxes to a personal security account
(PSA). The reason we suggest such a significant change relates to our
perceptions of the problems that have arisen under the current system
and to our belief that the solutions proposed by other Advisory Council members are not achievable. While there is consensus among all
council members that a portion of Social Security Trust Funds should
be invested in the capital base of our economy, only our proposal
would increase the level of national savings without creating pools of
savings so large that it would be impractical and undesirable to have
them invested in the private capital markets under the auspices of a
centrally managed fund.

The Problem of Financing

One popular notion about Social Security's financing status is that the
actuarial imbalances in the system are relatively minor. Holders of this
notion point to the *1995 Social Security Trustees Annual Report,*
which shows that the system is underfunded by only a projected 2.17
percent of covered payroll. While seemingly small—amounting to only

about 1.1 percent each for workers and employers—it is a significant and serious amount. In fact, the 2.17 percent actuarial deficit is largely a numerical artifact. It is calculated to give us a point-in-time estimate of the seventy-five-year relationship between Social Security's expected income and outlays. The 2.17 percent figure suggests that if we reduce future outlays by an average of 2.17 percent of covered payroll over the next seventy-five years, the system would have sufficient resources to pay benefits at reduced levels until 2070 or, alternatively, that if we raise payroll by 2.17 percent we could pay future benefits at the levels promised by current law. The problem is that neither of these options was attainable at the time the 2.17 percent was calculated (spring 1995). The subsequent delays in making the change will almost certainly require changes larger than the 2.17 percent deficit posted in 1995.

Intergenerational Equity and Social Security

In the past, Social Security Advisory Councils have focused on a concept of equity whereby workers who pay more into the system receive higher benefits. The present Advisory Council has focused on a broader concept of equity, namely on whether Social Security provides workers with a fair rate of return on their contributions into the system and whether it provides consistent treatment for various generations of workers. In the early years, for example, Social Security was an extremely good buy; an average wage worker who had never married and who retired at age sixty-five in 1960 could expect to receive benefits that were seven to nine times the value of lifetime payroll taxes paid on his or her wages accumulated with interest.

Over time, the relative value of lifetime benefits compared to lifetime contributions has declined, a trend that continues today. Indeed, workers today, paying the highest real taxes in the history of the program, are already facing the prospect of reduced benefits relative to those being provided to current retirees. Thus, for an average wage earner born in 1960 who is single or who is married to a spouse also earning average wages, the expected value of Social Security benefits under current law will be only be 75 to 90 percent of the value of the taxes paid on their lifetime earnings accumulated with interest. In short, the relationship between the accumulated payroll taxes that many workers are expected to pay and the Social Security benefits that they can expect to receive under the current structure is both unfair and unsustainable. In addition, there is growing evidence that lack of confidence in the system, momentarily halted by surplus buildups in the wake of the 1983 amendments, is on the rise again.

A Proposed Solution to the Social Security Financing Problem

One group of Social Security Advisory Council members put forward a Social Security reform plan that would create mandatory personal security accounts dedicated to retirement savings and financed by a rebate of a portion of the Federal Insurance Contribution Act (FICA) payroll tax. This option would allow us to restore Social Security to actuarial balance. It would ultimately raise the money's worth ratios for program participants and, thus, increase the perceptions of fairness in the program across generations. It would improve workers' perceptions about the security of their benefits, because a significant portion of their retirement security would be reflected in the value of financial assets that they could hold and control in their own name. This proposal could be implemented quickly enough that the benefit levels for the baby boom generation could largely be protected against substantial cutbacks. It would provide a vital pool of savings that would help to expand our economy so that the expected growth in the retiree population could be more easily sustained by a stable or shrinking workforce in the early twenty-first century.

Personal Security Accounts and Retirement Benefits

PSAs would hold a portion of the payroll tax that has traditionally been used to finance retirement benefits through Social Security. The annual contributions to the accounts would be equal to 5 percent of payroll, or approximately one-half of the current FICA payroll tax used to finance benefits for elderly retirees. PSAs would be subject to necessary regulatory restrictions to make sure they were invested in financial instruments widely available in the financial markets and that they were held for retirement purposes. While individuals could not withdraw funds until they had met age criteria qualifying them for benefits, PSAs would be under the sole direction of the workers who owned them. The young survivors and disability programs would continue to be financed and administered through Social Security.

Under this proposal, the half of the payroll tax that is not rebated to workers would continue to fund retirement benefits provided through Social Security. The current benefit structure would remain in place for individuals already retired and receiving Social Security benefits and for workers grandfathered under the existing system. During the transition period, individuals not grandfathered under the current system would receive a modified benefit; ultimately, however, the total benefits paid to retirees would come from the two separate tiers of the system. The first tier would be a basic flat-rate benefit provided through Social Security. For individuals with relatively full career earnings, this benefit would be roughly equal to $410 in 1996 dollars, indexed by the growth in average wages for future years. For individuals who do not work a full career, half of the flat benefits would be earned with ten years of covered earnings. For these individuals, additional benefits would be earned at a rate of 2 percent per year for which four quarters of covered earnings were reported. The second-tier benefit would be based on the balance in the PSA accumulated over a worker's career.

Also under this proposal, the normal retirement age would begin to increase in the year 2000 at a rate of two months per year until it reaches sixty-eight years of age in 2017. Beyond 2017, the normal retirement age would continue to increase at the rate of one month every other year, roughly the rate of increase in life expectancy among the elderly population as projected by Social Security actuaries. Congress would be required to make any necessary adjustments to ensure that this balance between life expectancy and the ability to extend individuals' working lives was maintained.

The implementation date for the transition to the new plan would be January 1, 1998. Workers age fifty-five or older would continue to be covered under the existing system and would pay taxes and receive benefits in accordance with current law, subject to retirement age and benefit taxation that would apply generally under the proposal. Individuals between ages twenty-five and fifty-five would receive a first-tier benefit under Social Security that is a combination of their accrued benefit under the existing system and a pro rata share of the flat benefit that would be provided under the new system. Their second tier would be the amount financed by the accumulated balance in the PSA. Workers under age twenty-five would be fully covered under the new system.

The Taxation of Benefits

Under this proposal, the taxation of Social Security benefits would be consistent with the tax treatment of retirement savings in tax-qualified plans. Employer contributions for benefits would continue to be deductible expenses, while employee contributions would continue to be made on a posttax basis. To the extent that benefits are financed by pretax dollars, they would be taxable at distribution. For people covered under the current system, 50 percent of benefits would be taxable. For people covered under the new system, we assume that employers' deductible contributions would be used to finance the first-tier benefit. Thus, these benefits would be taxable to the extent that they are financed by employer contributions. We assume employees' posttax contributions would finance the PSAs, and thus distributions from these accounts would be tax free.

Transition Financing

Under the PSA proposal, Social Security as we know it today would be transformed from a system largely funded on a pay-as-you-go basis to one that is significantly funded. One of the problems created by this shift is that previously accrued but unfunded liabilities continue to mature during the transition period at the same time that future benefits are being prefunded. In the specific case of this proposal, people who are currently retired or above age fifty-five would continue to receive benefits roughly in accordance with current law. However, many people between ages twenty-five and fifty-five would also receive larger benefits from Social Security than they would receive if they could be immediately moved into the flat-benefit system provided under the first tier of the modified plan. In this case, the benefit stream promised by current law would persist for a while and only then taper down, but the tax rebates for the PSAs would begin immediately. Additional funds, therefore, would be required to meet projected benefits during the transition.

There are several ways that the transition costs implied by this proposal could be financed. Of these alternatives, we suggest that they be paid by an explicit tax—dubbed a liberty tax, because it would free us over time from a completely unfunded retirement program (predicated entirely on the willingness and ability of younger workers and future generations to cover future liabilities) to a program that is significantly funded. Through PSAs, workers would accumulate rights to benefits based on their own savings and investments. This liberty tax could take several forms: a surtax on the regular income tax, a supplemental payroll tax, or a completely new tax levied independently of current sources of federal revenues.

Advocates of the PSA plan prefer a consumption tax as the mechanism to finance the transition costs incurred under the proposal, because it would create less of a drag on economic output than would a payroll tax. We also believe that a consumption tax would encourage saving, further encouraging economic growth. In the final recommendations, however, we propose that the transition be financed by an increase in the payroll tax. While we do so reluctantly, practical considerations motivated us to propose the increased payroll tax option. The consumption tax originally recommended would have been a 1 percent national sales tax. The problem with such a tax is that the federal government does not have the administrative machinery in place to collect such a tax and that it would be relatively inefficient to create a system to collect a relatively small tax of this sort. In addition, we were concerned about the potential interactions between a consumption tax and the existing federal income tax. We are quite clear, however, that, should the federal government move more generally toward a consumption tax system, adding on to such a tax would be preferable to our proposed payroll tax increase for financing the transition to a PSA system.

Either a 1.5 percent payroll tax or a 1 percent consumption sales tax would require that some of the statutory unfunded obligations of Social Security be converted into more formal debt over a portion of the transition period. The amount of that debt will undoubtedly be an important consideration in evaluating the merits of this overall proposal. Based on the intermediate assumptions of the Social Security actuaries for valuing Social Security, the Old Age, Survivors, and Disability Insurance (OASDI) Trust Funds, which would be used to finance outstanding liabilities under the old system as well as new liabilities for the flat benefit under the new system, OASDI would have a balance of $661 billion by the end of 1997. The balance would then start to decline as the modified system was implemented. By 2010, the trust funds would be depleted, by 2015 they would total $562 billion, and between 2045 and 2050 they would peak at just over $10 trillion nominal dollars ($1.2 trillion in 1996 dollars). Beyond 2050, the liberty bond balances would start to decline and would be fully paid off by 2070.

In the light of current budgetary debates, running up an additional $650 billion in federal debt may seem a bit outlandish. It is critical to keep in mind, however, that this accruing debt would simply be an explicit recognition of an implicit obligation that already exists under Social Security. The liberty tax could be thought of as taking out an explicit mortgage to help pay off a significant portion of the unfunded statutory obligations created over the past sixty years of the OASDI program. A seventy-year mortgage may seem like a long one, but if an individual can take out a thirty-year mortgage to buy a house, surely a country can take out a seventy-year mortgage, given the potential benefits.

PSAs as a Source of Capital

One important concern about the proposal is whether the PSA balances will represent new savings or whether they will merely displace other forms of savings. The economic literature is inconclusive on this question because of divergent conclusions about the effects of Social Security on private savings. These ambiguities notwithstanding, the reason for saving for retirement is to accumulate sufficient wealth during one's working career to support a standard of living in retirement that is roughly equivalent to that attained prior to retirement. Today, the overwhelming majority of retirement saving accomplished in this country is through accumulating Social Security and employer-sponsored retirement plans. One goal of the PSA plan is to accumulate individual retirement wealth for workers that is roughly akin to the retirement wealth they might accumulate under Social Security—but with one big difference. We would fund a portion of that wealth with real assets instead of pay-as-you-go obligations for future generations. If these goals were realized, they should result in the creation of real wealth that would not have otherwise been achieved. At the end of the transition to the plan outlined here, projected PSA balances would be 1.7 times gross domestic product—an amount that would equal about $11 trillion if we were there today.

Concerns about the PSA Proposal

Four other concerns have been raised about the PSA proposal: (1) support for the system will wither, especially among higher-wage workers, if the system is restructured into the two tiers that we suggest; (2) the proposal exposes workers to undue risk by allowing them to invest a portion of their own retirement assets; (3) many people are ignorant about investing; and (4) the proposal would create a financial bonanza for the business of asset management, and most of the return on retirement assets would be eaten up by the administrative costs associated with individual investing.

Support for Social Security in a Two-Tiered System   Social Security has always had two important goals: to provide retirees with an adequate income to sustain a decent life in retirement and to treat participants equitably. While these two goals have been muddled in the public's mind over the years, the muddling has been relatively noncontroversial because, until now, virtually all participants have gotten an actuarially good deal from the program. The divergent treatment of different generations suggests, however, that this situation is changing. The fundamental premise of the PSA proposal is that we should separate and clarify the two goals.

The adequacy goal under Social Security has led us to a program that redistributes income. In the PSA proposal, we are keeping the redistributional element of the system through the flat benefit that would be paid by Social Security. If we can convince the American people that it is desirable to create retirement income redistribution through a single-tiered system by means of a tilted benefit formula, why can't we convince them that similar redistribution is desirable through a two-tiered system?

The equity goal has led us to design a program that provides higher benefits for people making larger contributions. Looking to the future, however, Social Security provides such a low rate of return that many workers want to have alternative investment choices. Both of the other options being offered by other Advisory Council members concede this desire on the part of workers. The PSA proposal would give workers the opportunity to realize a fair rate of return on a significant portion of their mandatory retirement contribution.

Risk and Retirement Benefits for Future Generations   One common criticism of the PSA proposal is that it would expose workers to the risks of financial investing. This is clearly true. Yet, it is not clear that the risks posed by the financial markets are any greater than the political risks to which previously promised retirement benefits are now exposed or that this risk is not offset by the higher expected benefits of this option over the other options considered. The recent Medicare debate is instructive here on the question of risks in the long term. While most of the Advisory Council's attention has focused on how much to cut out of Medicare over the short term (seven years), there was no dissent from current defenders of the Medicare system (or anyone else) about convening a special commission to study how Medicare might be modified to deal with the baby boomers' claims on the system. This debate about how to address unfunded future liabilities must extend, as well, to Social Security.

While there is risk in investing accumulated wealth, there is even greater risk in not having any wealth to invest. Rather than depend on the future good faith of various third parties, owners of PSAs would have control over their personal interests even if future policy makers decide that prior governmental commitments cannot be met. To appreciate the relative size of financial versus political risks, consider the scenario of bringing Social Security back into actuarial balance purely through benefit reductions, a scenario seriously considered by the Advisory Council. In short, such an approach would have a greater impact on many middle-aged workers than if they had all of their retirement assets in the stock market in October 1987—a month that experienced the largest decline in the stock market since the crash of 1929.

People's Ignorance Requires Pooled Assets   While there is universal agreement among Advisory Council members that some retirement assets should be invested in private capital markets, there are several reasons not to pool Social Security investments in private markets—investments that, under one option, could amount to $1.5 trillion by 2010. Some Advisory Council members conjured up a hypothetical way to manage the pooled investment of Social Security assets in the private financial markets so as to insure against political influence in the investment decisions. The Advisory Council cannot, however, design a model that would bind Congress's ability—or that of any future Congress—to make new laws or amend old ones. The recent suggestions by Clinton administration policy makers in the Department of Labor that assets in employer-sponsored, defined-benefit plans should be invested in certain vehicles because of their social merit—rather than purely for the economic welfare of the participants of the plans— are an indication of the political temptation to put retirement assets to some use other than the security of workers.

The members of the Advisory Council supporting the PSA proposal concluded that the only effective way to expand the investment options for contributions to Social Security is through the establishment of truly individualized accounts.

Management and Administrative Issues   Other criticisms of PSAs center on the extremely high rates that investment managers might charge for managing the funds and on the possibility that unscrupulous fund managers would swindle workers out of the hard-earned contributions to their personal accounts. We believe that regulatory provisions—including licensure and limits on administrative fees—would eliminate most of the risk of fraud and abuse faced by funds being offered as PSA options. Furthermore, the widespread availability of mutual fund options with annual administrative fees well below 1 percent per year and increased competition for the management of the funds will limit these fees to reasonable levels.

Conclusion

There are three potential advantages to modifying the current Social Security system along the lines of the PSA model: (1) creating substantial wealth that would increasingly back the retirement security of U.S. workers, (2) generating benefit levels that significantly exceed those that can be offered by the current Social Security system or any of the alternatives considered by the Advisory Council, and (3) providing clearly superior value to many workers participating in the plan relative to the current system or any of the other alternatives being considered by the Advisory Council. This is especially the case for younger workers and for future workers. Given the burden that the baby boomers' retirement will place on younger and future workers, we must do everything possible to ensure that those workers enjoy a fair return on their own retirement savings. We must do everything to restore faith that participating in this system while they work will secure their welfare during their own retirement. PSAs are the answer.

11

Does Medicare Make Sense as an Age-Related Program?

MARILYN MOON

In the 1990s, Medicare and other public programs are facing unprecedented scrutiny by taxpayers who fear they are not getting full value for their dollars. And although Medicare consistently ranks among the most popular federal programs, in order to achieve the promises of politicians who wish to balance the budget while cutting taxes, few programs can be immune to major reductions. Moreover, legitimate concerns about the future of our entitlement programs and somewhat more gratuitous warnings about intergenerational warfare also dictate the need to carefully reexamine Medicare. It is in this context that a frank discussion about age-related programs is raised.

Context matters. Raising the question about the need for a separate age-related health care program in the midst of a serious debate about providing universal health insurance coverage for all Americans is quite different from raising the issue in the context of a discussion about what programs to eliminate or scale back. If the context is debate about achieving a program in which health insurance is available to everyone, then age appropriateness raises questions about the varying needs of populations of different ages. It also may evoke other distinctions, such as the mode of financing appropriate for various age groups.

Answers concerning the usefulness of Medicare in this context would be quite different from the answers emerging when evaluating whether Medicare, as the major non-means-tested health care program, should be scaled back substantially. Then the issue becomes one of whether preferential treatment for a particular age group is reasonable. In a world of scarce resources, which are the most deserving groups? Since the collapse of serious debate on universal coverage in 1994, Medicare's future is being discussed in this latter context.

But even in this political environment, it is important to consider whether singling out elderly people for a special health care program is appropriate. First, to understand the appropriate role of Medicare, it is important to examine it as a retirement program as well as an age-related one. In that sense, age is largely a proxy for retirement, and Medicare effectively extends insurance to people who are, in large part, out of the labor force and for whom group insurance is therefore difficult to obtain. Most Americans get their health care benefits through their employer or the employer of a family member. Such coverage is at least partially subsidized by the employer and, just as important, people obtain "group" insurance, which is more efficient to provide and considerably less expensive to buy than individually based policies. And, historically, few insurance companies have wanted to offer policies to people over age sixty-five. Not only are there expenses in marketing to individuals, but also older Americans were considered an undesirable risk group in the 1950s and early 1960s. While younger families were increasingly obtaining insurance, elderly people were left behind. The health care have-nots were, increasingly, older Americans. In large measure, government took on the task because of a failure of the market to offer such services.

Age also plays another positive role in insurance. Even under private coverage, people of different ages are recognized as having different needs and different levels of expenditures. For example, people over sixty-five in the United States spend about 3.8 times as much as younger persons do on health care (Lefkowitz and Monheit 1991). Thus, to some extent age distinctions may be a natural way to subdivide the population by risk group. Among those under age sixty-five, for example, insurance companies often set premiums based on age, and states that establish rules for acceptable variations in insurance usually include age as a legitimate factor. Medicare effectively groups together a population of those most expensive to insure.

Thus, it is possible to conclude that some age-related policies have outlived their usefulness while others, like Medicare, may still play an important role. What about the future? We are now at a point in which private insurers are beginning to rethink their earlier decision to avoid seniors, and at least some of them are expressing interest in taking on this part of the population. As yet, however, their willingness to serve elderly people has been tested only moderately. Supplemental insurance, for example, carries limited liabilities: Medicare bears more of a risk. Further, health maintenance organizations (HMOs) that are allowed to enroll Medicare beneficiaries still cover only a minority of older beneficiaries, and many believe they have been able to successfully avoid covering the sickest among this population (Brown et al. 1993).

At the same time, many employers who have offered subsidies for insurance before their retirees become eligible for Medicare and for Medicare supplemental benefits are now beginning to reduce their commitments. Although this has not yet had a major impact on the portion of individuals served by former employers, it certainly seems that retiree coverage has peaked (Mazo, Rappaport, and Schieber 1994). These two competing trends underscore the point that any consideration of the future of Medicare raises financing, insurance, and benefits issues, each of which is discussed below.

Financing Issues

When Medicare was enacted in 1965, one of the claims was that almost no one over the age of sixty-five could afford private insurance; they were simply too poor (Marmor 1970). While that was certainly never true for all of those over sixty-five, the low-income population was a much greater proportion of all elderly people than it is today. The greater average affluence of older Americans has caused some policy makers to question the need for Medicare as it currently stands. However, Medicare beneficiaries are now more heterogeneous than in the past. A large number still would need subsidies before they could purchase insurance, but many older couples, particularly, are now as well off as their younger counterparts—and better off than very young families (see, e.g., Moon and Ruggles 1994).

Consequently, one of the challenging issues for financing health care for older Americans is how best to recognize this heterogeneity in economic status. For some, the answer is simple: means-test the program and limit its availability to those who are unable to afford insurance on their own. If Medicare were to be stringently means tested, however, it might make more sense to combine it with a broader program for all families, thereby eliminating the age-related nature of the program. In fact, there would be little reason for retaining both Medicare and Medicaid—the public program that now serves low-income seniors as well as others. But Medicare might be retained with a somewhat more generous means test, while further scaling back Medicaid. In that case, making the benefit age related would still serve as a way of providing preferential treatment to one age group, while limiting further the liabilities that government faces in providing health care services. A second way in which age relating arises in the current debate over how to scale back federal spending is the question of the appropriate age for eligibility for Medicare. An alternative cost-saving approach to means testing is to raise the age of eligibility from sixty-five to sixty-eight or seventy, for example. The age relating of Medicare would remain but would also be used to further limit coverage.

Is age relating a good way of identifying and meeting the needs of Americans? Raising the age of eligibility would tend to retain benefits for those most in need. But, in fact, age is not a very good proxy for need. That is, the health status of people age sixty-five and older varies substantially within each age group (Helbing 1993). And spending also varies more within each age group than across groups. For example, although the oldest old do use more health care than other age groups among elderly people, the differential is not nearly as dramatic as many believe. Medicare's beneficiaries over age eighty-five represent 10 percent of enrollees and account for just 14 percent of total spending. Compare this to the fact that the top 10 percent of Medicare beneficiaries in terms of spending account for 70 percent of Medicare expenditures (U.S. Health Care Financing Administration 1995).

In addition, the ability to afford to insure against ill health also varies substantially within age groups. While younger members of the Medicare-eligible population tend to have higher incomes than their counterparts who are over eighty, averages hide a great deal of diversity within this population. If the justification is to focus more on the ability to pay, then an income or means test is certainly a more direct way to do so. But many supporters of Medicare do not want to see it make major distinctions in eligibility by income. The popularity of the program arises in part because of its universality, prompting some to argue that universality should simply begin a little later. However, this is a very crude mechanism if done to serve as a proxy for targeting Medicare by ability to pay.

A second justification for raising the eligibility age arises over the longer life expectancies of older Americans. People who turned sixty-five in 1995 will live longer than those who turned sixty-five in 1965, at Medicare's inception (U.S. Bureau of the Census 1994). The higher costs of such additional years of coverage must be paid for in some way, and when these are combined with pressures that will arise from the aging of the baby boom generation, some changes will need to be made. In the eyes of many, that means delaying eligibility by raising the age at which people qualify for Medicare. A slow phase-in of that change would coincide with the rising burdens that demography will pose. Thus, it might be argued on grounds of intergenerational equity to fund only a given number of years at the end of life.

Indeed, the arguments posed by supporters of this approach often draw analogies to Social Security, where the normal age of retirement is scheduled to begin rising in the year 2000. It will eventually reach sixty-seven, and future policy changes in this program are likely to move that age even higher. But several things are quite different for Medicare. First, while the normal age of eligibility would rise for Social Security, under current law people could still choose to draw benefits at age sixty-two. They would simply receive a smaller benefit. Medicare, on the other hand, as now constituted does not offer an early eligibility option. Further, the problems discussed in the next section concerning sharing of risks in insurance and the lack of access to reasonable coverage in the private sector also need to be taken into account.

Despite these potential problems, it seems likely that increasing the age of eligibility for Medicare will be seriously debated in the near future. In fact, it was part of the savings plan offered by the U.S. Senate but then omitted from the final proposal in the Balanced Budget Act of 1995, which President Clinton vetoed. Since 1997 and beyond will likely see even more dramatic savings proposals for Medicare, increasing the age of eligibility is likely to continue to be on the agenda. Further, when it is debated as part of a broader package of budget savings, this change in Medicare may be preferred to more stringent means testing or other types of changes, such as moving Medicare to a voucher-type system.

One way to soften the blow of an increase in the age of eligibility for Medicare might be to create a new standard for qualifying for disability above a certain age. In that case, at least those who were not able to work longer because of health problems could still get

Medicare as disabled beneficiaries even if they did not yet qualify on the basis of the new age criteria. Similarly, eligibility for Medicaid could be expanded somewhat for those who might be disenfranchised by a higher age of receipt for Medicare. And finally, absent broad insurance reform, it would be crucial to allow older Americans to buy into the program, since they otherwise might not be able to attain insurance at any price.

Insurance Issues

Affordability and how to pay for insurance are not the only issues surrounding the appropriateness of an age-based public health insurance program. Medicare also raises questions concerning the very nature of health insurance protection. For example, one of Medicare's strengths is its sharing of risks across a large group of the population. With about thirty-eight million beneficiaries, Medicare is essentially the largest risk group for health insurance in the United States. Implicitly, costs for eighty-five-year-olds with health problems are averaged with costs for healthy seventy-year-olds, making insurance less expensive than if these eighty-five-year-olds were seeking insurance in the private market from a company that covered a much smaller number of people.

But if this pooling of risk is such a good idea for an elderly and disabled population, what about an insurance pool of all Americans? In that case, risks would be pooled to the greatest extent possible. Indeed, this was a goal of many advocates of national health insurance. Such an approach would work, however, only with an agreement across all generations that such pooling should take place, and it most likely needs a governmental mechanism to finance one large health plan. This is because total community rating—that is, setting only one price for health insurance—is essentially a very redistributive system at any one point in time. Because older people tend to require more health care, establishing a single insurance premium in a given area would require most young people to pay much more than the costs of their own care for their coverage. Older persons, on the other hand, would pay much less. And since younger families tend to be less well off, such impacts raise equity issues. Recognizing this, all the health reform plans of 1994—except the fully tax-financed single-payer plan—would have kept Medicare separate from the rest of the system to limit the full extent of community rating. (And some plans would have allowed some age distinctions within the under-sixty-five population, as well.)

Further, in our fragmented health care system, such community rating poses a number of problems. While there is some pressure to reform insurance so that it is priced on the basis of at least a modified community-rated system, it would become much more difficult to do so if elderly and disabled persons are included as well as persons from birth through age sixty-four. For example, employers would be less likely to offer insurance to all workers if their rates were subsidizing the oldest old in our society as well. This would immediately raise the costs of insurance for such employers. (And there are the practical difficulties of applying full community rating in the United States, since, for example, employers can serve as their own insurers and restrict their risks to their own pool of workers.) Thus, for practical reasons, it makes sense to retain an age-related health insurance scheme for older people when there is no feasible way to deal with the redistributional questions that community rating raises in a decentralized insurance world.

This insurance issue also has implications for proposals to raise the age of eligibility for Medicare. Although younger elderly people—for example, those age sixty-five through seventy-four—have lower medical expenses than the oldest old, their expenses are still higher on average than those for the rest of the population. Consequently, raising the age of eligibility for Medicare would also have insurance consequences for the private system. How easy would it be for those in their sixties to obtain insurance through the private marketplace, for example? Employer-subsidized retiree benefits are still available to only a minority of retirees, so many people would have to purchase care through the individual insurance market. For younger people, individual insurance tends to be more expensive and come with more restrictions than group insurance; it might be even more difficult for individuals over sixty-five to obtain coverage.

At a minimum, private insurance reforms would be needed, but that would not overcome the affordability problem if they were priced at a very high level. For example, it would be important to have reforms that guarantee that people could obtain insurance and that limit restrictions, such as exclusions for preexisting conditions. But such reforms tend to raise the costs of insurance by ensuring that even those with health problems are not excluded from coverage. Alternatively, people could remain eligible for Medicare but could be required to pay more for such coverage—perhaps the full actuarial cost. Even so, it is likely that the numbers of uninsured persons would rise if Medicare is scaled back to begin at a later age.

In addition, proposals to fully or partially rely on private plans to cover Medicare beneficiaries can face very similar issues, particularly if Medicare offers its beneficiaries vouchers with set dollar amounts and then lets plans decide what they will actually charge beneficiaries. In such a defined-contribution world, Medicare would guarantee only a contribution rather than a basic benefit package, as is now the case. Beneficiaries would often have to supplement the Medicare voucher to buy a desired insurance plan. And when plans can charge additional premiums (as is now allowed to a limited degree under the HMO option and would have been allowed under the Balanced Budget Act of 1995), they could begin to influence even more dramatically who will enroll. For example, some might use high premiums to concentrate on a higher-income market. This would implicitly discriminate against older beneficiaries, who tend to have lower incomes. Moreover, by choosing what additional benefits to offer, plans may also discourage those beneficiaries who need home health care, for example, versus health club memberships.

An even further dilemma occurs for the rules that Medicare might establish. The voucher amount presumably would vary by the age and other circumstances of the beneficiary (as is now the case under the HMO option). But what requirements should be placed on the extra premium that plans charge beneficiaries? If it is required to be the same for all enrollees as under the current optional system, plans have little incentive to offer benefits or terms that will be attractive to older, sicker beneficiaries. But if plans are allowed to age rate their premiums, older beneficiaries may not be able to afford to join. Such options run the risk of implicitly discriminating against older beneficiaries, and moves in this direction need to be carefully studied.

Benefits Issues

Yet another issue concerning age-related benefits has to do with the appropriateness of the coverage offered to different types of individuals. For example, Medicare does not need to offer well-baby care in its package, but it could usefully recognize the higher likelihood of chronic disease and other problems faced by older people. Indeed, by having a separate program for aged and disabled persons, it should be possible to tailor benefits to the specific needs of this population. In practice, however, this potential advantage for Medicare has not come to pass.

When Medicare was established in 1965, a major concern was that it be viewed as a mainstream program attractive to beneficiaries and providers of care (Moon 1993). Consequently, efforts were made to have the program look much like insurance for younger families. Moreover, at least in the early 1960s, hospital care was viewed as the major health care access problem for elderly people. The lack of acute-care coverage for elders dominated the debate. Long-term care was considered a secondary issue. Criticism of Medicare's lack of support for chronic illness and long-term care is essentially an indirect compliment to the program for how well it has solved the problems of access to standard services for acute illness. But it is true that cost sharing is higher for those who have only ambulatory care needs, like multiple doctors' visits. And long-term care is technically not covered at all. In practice, the coverage of home health and skilled nursing care have moved Medicare more toward long-term care than was the case in the early years of the program, but many areas of need still go largely uncovered.

Could Medicare be improved in these additional areas? Certainly. But such expansions would be expensive, and the current political environment means that even maintaining existing service and eligibility levels will be difficult. Financing an expansion of covered services would likely require either greater beneficiary contributions into Medicare or a contraction of the eligible population. Higher premiums or cost sharing are certainly among the options now under consideration (although the savings would not be used to expand Medicare to other areas).

Medicare now allows individuals to opt for private HMO plans, which may offer additional services such as much lower cost sharing, preventive medicine, and especially prescription drug coverage. In exchange, beneficiaries agree to get all of their services from the HMO's doctors, hospitals, and other facilities. And while these plans may appeal to the very old, they are more appealing to younger beneficiaries. As yet, HMOs have not aggressively marketed to chronically ill persons or to other groups by offering benefits for special needs. Moreover, since some studies show that these plans do little to save money for the Medicare program, Medicare's payments to these plans will grow more slowly over time, which may limit the services they offer.

What about raising the age of eligibility and using some of the savings to expand help for the chronically ill and the disabled? Changes in Medicare's benefit package toward long-term care would make more sense if the program were targeted toward those age seventy-five and older. Certainly, for many older Americans up to age seventy-five, but even after that, acute health care spending remains very important: part of Medicare's financial problems stems from the rapid growth of heart bypass surgeries, hip replacements, cataract surgeries, and the like, which are performed on an ever-older population. A modified package of benefits, which would include long-term care for chronic illness, could be extended to the old old (age seventy or seventy-five, for example) and to the disabled, while offering a more basic plan with higher personal contributions to those below the new eligibility age. And this lower tier might be extended even further down the age scale to aid early retirees and perhaps even unburden some employers who now face high subsidy costs. This type of change could improve on basic proposals to raise the age of eligibility for Medicare. But it is hard to imagine how to design a package that would not raise overall costs—and that constraint is likely to foreclose any promising moves in this area.

Conclusion

The tenor of the debate regarding health care has changed immensely since May 1994. Prospects for expanding coverage under Medicare along with a minimal expansion of long-term-care services seemed plausible early in 1994. By the beginning of 1995, the discussion shifted to how much can be wrung out of the Medicare program to help balance the federal budget. While no legislation has passed, this emphasis on scaling back the program remains. And, even if Medicare were separated from the budget discussion, the future demographics and the strains they will place on public spending mean that we must take seriously the need to streamline this program.

Thus, with substantial reductions in federal spending on the horizon for the Medicare program, some new ways of thinking about the program are needed. Rather than rejecting a proposal such as raising the age of eligibility as undesirable, we must view it in the context of other possible changes. How does such a proposal measure up to means-testing the program or converting it to a voucher system? These and other proposals for change have both crude and subtle impacts on

Americans of different ages. Vouchers, for example, are likely to be harder on the oldest old, while means testing eliminates higher-income persons of any age. But how do we weigh these alternatives in the context of an individual's lifetime? These alternatives need careful debate before any are adopted.

In this new environment, the questioning of age-related programs takes on a very different meaning from in the past, when universal health insurance seemed a possibility. Instead, we are more likely to retain Medicare as an age-related program, although the ages affected are likely to change over time. Age is a simple criterion to measure and enforce—as compared to economic resources or levels of disability, for example. A higher eligibility age can also be viewed as consistent with the expanding life expectancies of older Americans, so Medicare continues to cover people for an average fixed number of years at the end of life. These basic factors may make this policy preferable to other changes.

There are also legitimate insurance reasons to maintain age distinctions. To keep insurance more affordable for younger people, it is appropriate to have a separate program for elders, like Medicare. An age-defined program also allows fine-tuning of coverage, although Medicare has not taken advantage of this opportunity and it may now be too expensive to change, at least in the current political climate.

But if raising the age of eligibility for Medicare is the direction in which we move, it will be critical to push other parts of society to develop consistent policies and attitudes. First, Social Security and Medicare need to be closely coordinated. If reductions in benefits occur for both by, for example, raising the age of eligibility, those who must retire early will find it very expensive to both subsist on reduced Social Security benefits and seek their own health insurance. But even more important, private pensions, work opportunities for older workers, rules for private insurance, and the general attitudes of society must also change if higher age criteria are to be successful and not simply result in lower standards of living over time.

Acknowledgments

The author would like to acknowledge the Henry J. Kaiser Family Foundation for funding for the article on which this chapter is based (it appeared in *Generations*) and the Commonwealth Fund's Program on Medicare's Future for funding for the revisions.

References

Brown, R., D. Clement, J. Hill, S. Rettchin, and J. Bergeron. 1993. Do Health Maintenance Organizations Work for Medicare? *Health Care Financing Review* 15:7–23.

Helbing, C. 1993. Medicare Program Expenditures. *Health Care Financing Review: Annual Statistical Supplement, 1992.* Washington, D.C.: Government Printing Office.

Lefkowitz, D., and A. Monheit. 1991. Health Insurance, Use of Health Services, and Healthcare Expenditures. *National Medical Expenditure Survey Research Findings 12.* Publication 92–0017. Rockville, Md.: U.S. Public Health Service, Agency for Health Care Policy and Research.

Marmor, T. 1970. *The Politics of Medicare.* Chicago: Aldine.

Mazo, J., A. Rappaport, and S. Schieber. 1994. *Providing Health Care Benefits in Retirement.* Philadelphia: Pension Research Council and University of Pennsylvania Press.

Moon, M. 1993. *Medicare Now and in the Future.* Washington, D.C.: Urban Institute.

Moon, M., and P. Ruggles. 1994. The Needy or the Greedy? Assessing the Income Support Needs of an Aging Population. In T. Marmor, T. Smeeding, and V. Greene, eds., *Economic Security and Intergenerational Justice: A Look at North America.* Washington, D.C.: Urban Institute.

U.S. Bureau of the Census. 1994. *Statistical Abstract of the United States, 1994.* Washington, D.C.: Government Printing Office.

U.S. Health Care Financing Administration. 1995. *Health Care Financing Review Medicare and Medicaid Statistical Supplement.* Baltimore: U.S. Department of Health and Human Services.

12

Medicaid
*The Shifting Place of Old People in a
Needs-Based Health Program*

ELIZABETH A. KUTZA

While Medicare dominates discussion as regards health care and the elderly, the importance of Medicaid to older people should not be underestimated. Medicaid (Title XIX of the Social Security Act), which passed at the same time as Medicare in 1965, is substantially different in its administrative details and its financing. Unlike Medicare, which operates much like a private health insurance program for individuals who are elderly or disabled, Medicaid is a grant-in-aid program that helps states pay for medical assistance for certain individuals and families with low income and few resources. Both are entitlement programs, but in one entitlement rests on age and contributions through covered employment, while in the other it rests on low-income status.

Funding for Medicare comes from payroll tax contributions, premiums, and cost-sharing payments; funding for Medicaid comes from general revenues at both the federal and the state level. While funding is shared by the federal and state governments, the states have wide latitude in establishing Medicaid eligibility standards, type and scope of services, and rate of payment to providers. As a result, the Medicaid program varies considerably from state to state. Total outlays for the Medicaid program were $135.4 billion for 1994 ($78.1 billion in federal and $57.3 billion in state funds), which includes vendor payments and administrative costs (U.S. Social Security Administration 1995). Of the 35,056 recipients receiving Medicaid benefits in 1994, 70 percent were either poor children (under twenty-one years of age) or their parents.

Under federal guidelines, some elderly people—those who are receiving federal Supplemental Security Income (SSI) cash benefits—must be covered under the Medicaid program. SSI is a federal program that provides income support to elderly persons whose incomes fall below a nationally designated standard. In 1995, the federal SSI benefit rate for an elderly individual living in her own household with no other countable income was $458 a month; for a couple with both husband and wife eligible, the SSI benefit rate was $687 a month. States have the option of covering other categorically needy groups, including (1) older people who have incomes above SSI eligibility but below the federal poverty guidelines, and (2) those institutionalized individuals with incomes and resources below specified limits. Finally, states also have the option of extending eligibility to those who are "medically needy," that is, those who have too much income to qualify under the mandatory or optional categorically needy levels. This option allows the individuals to "spend down" to Medicaid eligibility. This has been an especially important source of funding for middle-class older Americans who are institutionalized in nursing facilities.

Another way that the Medicaid program serves older people is through its relationship to the Medicare program. While people who have insured status under Social Security receive Medicare hospital insurance benefits automatically, they must pay a monthly premium for coverage under Medicare's supplemental medical insurance provisions. The state Medicaid agency may pay those premiums for Medicaid recipients entitled to Medicare. For certain "qualified Medicare beneficiaries" (those Medicare-entitled people with resources at or below twice the standard allowed under the SSI program and with incomes below the federal poverty guidelines), the state pays all the premiums and cost-sharing expenses for hospital insurance and supplemental medical insurance.

Altogether, those provisions in 1994 allowed 4.04 million persons age sixty-five or older to participate in the Medicaid program. With older people representing 11.5 percent of all beneficiaries, vendor payments on behalf of this age group totaled $33.4 billion in 1994, or 30.9 percent of the total outlays. Disabled people, too, receive substantial benefit from Medicaid. They represent 15.3 percent of beneficiaries and 38.5 percent of the total vendor payments (U.S. Social Security Administration 1995). A look at vendor payments by type of

Table 12.1.
Distribution of Medicaid Payments by Type of Medical Service,
Fiscal Year 1991 (in percentages)

Medical Service	Aged	Disabled
Nursing facilities	67.3	12.4
Intermediate care facilities for the mentally retarded	1.7	25.4
Inpatient hospital	6.4	26.0
Home health	8.0	6.8
Other	16.6	29.4

medical service shows distinctions between these two groups, however. Table 12.1 displays these differences.

The dominant benefit under Medicaid for older people is for the payment of nursing facility care. For disabled people, institutional care both in nursing facilities and in intermediate care facilities for the mentally retarded represents over one-third of expenditures, followed by inpatient hospital care (a benefit that Medicare provides for aged persons) and other medical expenses (e.g., physician and other provider services, outpatient care, and laboratory and drug expenses).

Thus, the importance of Medicaid to both poor and medically needy aged persons is clear. They rely on it as a supplement to Medicare and a significant source of funding for nursing home care.

Current Issues in Medicaid

Medicaid's success in increasing access to medical and long-term care services has resulted in concerns about its increasing costs. States, especially, are facing challenges in meeting their growing Medicaid financial responsibilities. At the same time that Congress mandated expansion of the program in the late 1980s, the nation entered a recession that caused state revenues to decline. The impact of these two concurrent actions is shown in expenditure data. Payments to vendors in the Medicaid program rose from $5.1 billion in 1970 to $112.8 billion in 1994, an average annual growth rate of 14.7 percent. From 1989 to 1992, however, Medicaid outpaced total health care spending, increasing at an average annual rate of 20.5 percent (U.S. Health Care Financing Administration 1995).

Several factors contributed to this growth in spending. Coughlin, Ku, and Holahan (1994) attribute 36 percent to enrollment increases,

26 percent to medical care price inflation, and 33 percent to use and reimbursement above inflation. In addition, this recent spurt in spending can be attributed to what the Health Care Financing Administration (HCFA) calls "creative financing techniques" implemented by the states. These include the solicitation of voluntary donations from hospitals, the imposition of provider taxes on certain health care services, and an increase of payments to disproportionate-share hospitals (DSHs; i.e., hospitals serving a disproportionate share of low-income patients). The first two strategies can increase outlays without burden on either the federal or the state treasury, while the latter strategy allows states to leverage greater federal contributions to Medicaid. As Coughlin, Ku, and Holahan (1994, 152) point out, "These programs, virtually nonexistent in the mid-1980s, exploded in size between 1990 and 1992. By 1992, $7.8 billion was collected in provider taxes and donations, and intergovernmental transfers and DSH payments reached $17.4 billion." Opportunities for states to engage in these "creative financing techniques" declined, however, when Congress passed the Medicaid Voluntary Contributions and Provider-Specific Tax Amendments of 1991, a bill that greatly limited the states' use of special financing programs.

But concerns about the rapid growth of expenditures in the Medicaid program continue to generate calls for reform at national and state levels. Slowing the growth rate of Medicaid spending is seen as an important component in any effort to balance the federal budget. And because Medicaid now accounts for over 14 percent of states' expenditures from their general funds, it is also a major priority for the states, which on average finance 43 percent of Medicaid spending. As a recent U.S. Congressional Budget Office report (1996, 433) notes, "The emphasis on curtailing Medicaid expenditures represents a distinct change in philosophy from the late 1980s, when the priorities of the program were to expand eligibility and coverage."

In 1995, several proposals for reform surfaced in Washington, D.C., from a number of sources—the Congress, the president, the National Governors Association, and the Congressional Budget Office. The bill ultimately passed by Congress (but vetoed by President Clinton) would have converted Medicaid from an open-ended entitlement program (i.e., in which federal expenditures must meet the costs associated with every eligible beneficiary) with a mandated service package to a block grant (MediGrant) with few national standards. Federal expenditures for Medicaid would have been capped at some absolute limit and indexed far below the expected rate of growth. Holahan and Liska (1995) estimate that federal Medicaid expenditures would have been 28 percent below what would be expected under current law by the year 2002, while the Congressional Budget Office estimates that there would have been a 23 percent decline. While qualified Medicare beneficiaries and the elderly and disabled persons who meet SSI eligibility standards would have retained benefits under the MediGrant proposal, it appears that low-income elderly persons now covered at the option of a state by virtue of spend-down or medically needy provisions would have been excluded (Davis 1996).

President Clinton's proposal retained the entitlement nature of Medicaid but would have established limits per beneficiary on the growth of federal expenditures. While not abandoning federal standards, the president would have given states greater flexibility in contracting with managed care organizations, setting reimbursement rates, and organizing long-term care services. Under current law, the average spending for an elderly Medicaid beneficiary is expected to grow at an average annual rate of 6.9 percent. With a per capita cap, this rate of growth would have slowed to 4.3 percent (U.S. Congressional Budget Office 1996).

As Wiener (1996, 1) notes, "The [Medicaid] policy debate begins and ends with the notion that if states are given enough flexibility, they will figure out how to reduce the rate of growth in expenditures without hurting beneficiaries." The only evidence currently available as to whether this "notion" has merit is found in the experience of states that have tried to reform their own Medicaid systems under federal waiver authority.

Needs-Based Programs and Aged People

In the debate surrounding age versus need as a criterion for benefit eligibility, it is often asserted that needs-based programs will stigmatize older people and place them at a disadvantage. Whether this is the case in large part depends upon how *need* is defined. Typically, in U.S. social policy, need is defined as financial need and is determined by income and asset eligibility standards. Such standards, or means tests, can serve one of two functions: they can screen clients in or out of a service program, or they can be taken into consideration in the cost-sharing arrangements made with clients once they are accepted for the service. Most discussion around needs-based programs focuses on means tests used in the first way.

Under Medicaid, for example, income and asset standards determine the eligibility for subsidized health care services. Not all poor people are eligible for Medicaid, just those whose income and assets fall below a certain level. Because states can set these eligibility levels, the levels frequently are quite restrictive; income eligibility levels in most states are below the federally designated poverty level. Maximum countable assets in most states (i.e., the level of assets above which one is *ineligible* for the program) is $2,000. In addition to setting up monetary levels of eligibility, rule makers using means tests for eligibility also must deal with issues of the unit to be measured (individual or family) and the accounting period to be used.

Part of the objection to means-tested programs rests on equity considerations, that is, on issues of fairness. However, advocates for the elderly also object to means-tested programs because of the stigma associated with the receipt of benefits. Declaring oneself to be impoverished in order to receive benefits from a program like Medicaid is assumed to be demeaning to the individual. But in programs that provide health or social services, need can be defined as "need for service"—for example, illness, in the case of a health service; functional disability, in the case of a long-term care service. In such a scenario, income and asset rules can be avoided, and rules that essentially provide for cost sharing can be implemented. Such a system is more equitable among individuals, because public support for service is based on need for service, qualified by the individual's ability to share in those costs. Cost sharing is also less stigmatizing for beneficiaries.

Two policy initiatives proposed such a change in our long-term care system but were given very scant hearing in Congress. In 1990, the U.S. Bipartisan Commission on Comprehensive Health Care, more commonly referred to as the Pepper Commission, made its report, *Access to Health Care and Long-Term Care for All Americans*. The report recommends a social insurance program for home and community care under which eligibility would be determined by functional status, not age or income. Cost sharing was to be required, but generous income and asset protection also was to be in place. For example, full protection of income and assets was proposed for all nursing home users during the first three months of care. Three years later, President Clinton put forward his American Health Security Act, which also recommended a new long-term care program. As in the

Pepper Commission proposal, eligibility for services was based on functional status, not on income or age. Eligible individuals were expected to pay a coinsurance amount, according to a sliding scale, to cover a portion of the cost of the services they received.

Neither of these proposals was enacted, however, because universal entitlement proposals that base the receipt of service on need are a departure from our current approach of either categorical or means-tested eligibility. For that reason, they have not succeeded in the political marketplace.

Equity Considerations in the Definition of Need

Of course, moving away from means-tested eligibility standards to need-for-service eligibility standards in public programs does not exempt us from concerns about equity; it only presents us with different equity considerations depending on how "need for service" is defined. In the two examples cited above, need would have been defined in eligibility rules as a need for hands-on or supervisory assistance with three out of five activities of daily living or severe cognitive or mental impairment. By these criteria, many elderly persons would qualify for service. But perhaps a clearer illustration of the equity challenges faced by shifting criteria of need is a recent policy change in the state of Oregon.

In 1987, Oregon legislators faced with budget constraints decided not to pay for transplants for Medicaid patients but instead to fund basic health care and other social services. The public became aware of the trade-off with the death of a seven-year-old boy who otherwise might have been eligible for a state-financed transplant. Despite considerable public and media pressure, the lawmakers kept to their earlier legislative decision, but the case was the foundation for significant health care reform.

During its 1989 and 1991 sessions (Oregon has a biennial legislative session), the Oregon legislature passed six laws that began incremental reform of the health care system. The most widely publicized was Senate Bill 27 (1989), which extended Medicaid coverage to every Oregonian with income below the federal poverty level and provided a basic benefit package. Senate Bill 27 also created the Oregon Health Services Commission to rank medical services from most to least important for the entire population. The 1989 reforms also included bills that would require employers to cover all "permanent" employees and their dependents and a bill to fund the Oregon Medical Insurance Pool, which offers health insurance to people who cannot buy conventional coverage because of preexisting medical problems. In 1991, other bills created the Small Carrier Advisory Committee to design a basic benefit package for small businesses and required the Health Services Commission to integrate mental health and chemical dependency services into future priority lists as well as to begin offering the standard benefit package to seniors and persons with disabilities. Essentially, the Oregon health plan attempts to respond to the estimated 450,000 Oregonians not covered by any health plan.

What captured national attention was Senate Bill 27 and its priority ranking of services—"rationing," as it was called in the media. From the state's point of view, however, Senate Bill 27 provided for a process to develop a social and political consensus on what an "adequate," or "basic," package of benefits was to be. The bill established an eleven-member Health Services Commission made up of consumers and providers who, through a very public and open process, were to prioritize health care services from the most important to the least important based on the beneficial effect each service has on the entire population being served, as opposed to an individual within that population. Panels of medical experts looked at the medical effectiveness of each treatment intervention to maintain life. A series of public meetings and community forums solicited expressions of community values regarding health care. Oregonians said they wanted healthy mothers and babies, comfort care, and general preventive services. Prevention was ranked higher than treatment. Oregonians considered as less important treatment for conditions that get better on their own, cosmetic services, and experimental services.

All of these inputs ultimately led to a list of 688 "condition/ treatment pairs," which were grouped into seventeen categories and three groupings. Categories 1–9 were considered essential services, 10–13 were very important, and 14–17 were services valuable to certain individuals. After the list was generated, actuarial costs of each intervention were computed. The state legislature, which had no power to alter any ranking, then examined how much money was available under the Medicaid program and established a cutoff point of affordability. The state said that, of the 688 conditions on the list, only 568 could be afforded in the following biennium. Each biennium, the cutoff would be reconsidered in the light of available resources. Treatment for all conditions that ranked below the cutoff would not be reimbursed. For the most part, these were conditions for which treatment was considered ineffective, in which the condition would run its course regardless of treatment, or which were considered cosmetic.

In early 1995, older people and people with disabilities began to be enrolled in the Oregon Health Plan. In anticipation of this enrollment, the Oregon Health Services Commission began examining the list of condition/treatment pairs to see whether need, as defined by the list, was responsive to the needs of elderly persons. The exercise has provided a living example of the equity considerations that face policy makers even if need for service is used as an eligibility criterion. Many diseases that elderly persons experience were already ranked quite high (e.g., eye diseases, cancers). But some common conditions were not. An example of conditions not ranked high but subsequently reconsidered were those resulting from relaxation of the sphincter muscle (i.e., incontinence or impaction). Clearly, these conditions affect elderly and disabled persons more than other people.

Perhaps most interesting was the addition of five "dysfunction lines" that were to be considered along with the condition/treatment pairings: (1) respiration, eating, or elimination, (2) posture and movement, (3) respite care, (4) communication, and (5) chronic mental illness or dementias. Thus, for the treatment of a person with Alzheimer's disease, payment would be allowed for respite of a caregiver to compensate for the dysfunction associated with the disease. Similarly, the dysfunction lines allowed for equity among conditions that are frequently not considered equitably in health insurance plans. For example, if a person uses a wheelchair because of a stroke, insurance usually fully covers the person's care needs, but if a person uses a wheelchair because of a birth defect like cerebral palsy, the person frequently is not covered. Under the Oregon Health Plan, consideration under the dysfunction line of posture and movement makes the cerebral palsy patient eligible for the same ancillary services that a person with a stroke may have.

Enrollment of elderly and disabled persons in the Oregon Health Plan is now complete. But continuing to guarantee access to care for these high-cost patients is meeting with some challenges. A recent report on the health care market in Oregon's major metropolitan area, Portland, notes that the continued viability of the Oregon Health Plan's managed care coverage will depend on the financial commitment of state government and its support of managed care policy. Given the tight budgets in Oregon, brought on by the combined pressure of property tax limitation measures and competition for scarce state revenues by public safety and education advocates, reimbursement levels under the Oregon Health Plan are low. In 1993, for example, the ratio of Oregon's Medicaid maximum fees to the new Medicare fee schedule levels for physician services was 0.65 and for hospital visits was 0.63 (Winterbottom, Liska, and Obermaier 1995). As a result, the participation of managed care plans in the Oregon Health Plan declined. While the remaining plans have stepped in to fill the breach, there is concern as to what will happen if too many plans opt out of serving the Medicaid population.

On a more positive note, some managed care providers are beginning to work with Oregon's Senior and Disabled Services Division to better integrate the services of those Medicaid elderly persons who receive primary health care from a managed care plan and long-term care from the state's long-term care system. Public policy makers in Oregon are familiar with such an integrated service package, because Portland is the site of two national demonstrations: a social/health maintenance organization (S/HMO) and an On Lok replication called ElderPlace. Both are capitated systems that provide frail elderly persons with their primary care coverage and long-term services. The programs negotiate with the federal government for a capitated Medicare fee and with the state for a capitated Medicaid fee, the combined amount of which the provider uses to purchase services across the health care continuum. Based on the success of these demonstrations to reduce hospital utilization and to offer a "seamless" web of services for enrolled elderly persons, two area agencies on aging in the Portland metropolitan area (agencies that control long-term care dollars) are exploring ways to form alliances with managed health care providers who serve their clients. While the outcomes of these conversations are not yet clear, their direction is hopeful. As long as Medicaid remains a program that serves only poor people, however, such well-integrated services will be available for only a few elderly persons.

Conclusion

Medicaid is important to elderly people, especially those who need long-term care. The outcomes of the reform measures now under discussion in Washington and in the states are unclear. If cost containment measures such as block grants and per capita expenditure caps are put in place, elderly beneficiaries (who receive higher per capita benefits) may be hurt. States also may restrict coverage for the medically needy, further disadvantaging those elderly persons who rely on Medicaid for long-term care coverage.

Since absent among these discussions is any proposal to absorb Medicaid into a more universal health care or long-term care program, any change in the Medicaid program will leave the program's basic structure as a means-tested program in place. Its benefits, while serving many elderly persons, will be based not on age but on need for health care qualified by an income and asset test. These reforms may change the debate around access under the program, but the issues of equity will remain unchanged.

All programs require rules of participation and eligibility. Critics of eligibility rules that are means tested, like those in Medicaid, cite equity considerations as paramount. Unfortunately, such critics also frequently imply that these equity considerations are the exclusive domain of selective programs. In fact, concern for fairness among program participants like the elderly does not disappear if the rules are based on a need standard other than financial. The Oregon example shows how programs like Medicaid can remain sensitive to fairness issues as they refer to the special needs of older people and alerts us to the fact that, irrespective of the need standard used, we must always remain vigilant to the special circumstances that aging brings to the lives of individuals.

References

Coughlin, T., L. Ku, and J. Holahan. 1994. *Medicaid since 1980*. Washington, D.C.: Urban Institute.

Davis, K. 1996. *Medicaid: The Health Safety Net for the Nation's Poor.* New York: Commonwealth Fund.

Holahan, J., and D. Liska. 1995. *The Impact of the House and Senate Budget Committees Proposals on Medicaid Expenditures.* Washington, D.C.: Kaiser Commission on the Future of Medicaid.

U.S. Bipartisan Commission on Comprehensive Health Care. 1990. *Access to Health Care and Long-Term Care for All Americans.* Washington, D.C.: Government Printing Office.

U.S. Congressional Budget Office. 1996. *Reducing the Deficit: Spending and Revenue Options.* Washington, D.C.: Government Printing Office.

U.S. Health Care Financing Administration. 1995. *Health Care Financing Review: 1995 Statistical Supplement.* Washington, D.C.: Government Printing Office.

U.S. Social Security Administration. 1994. *Annual Statistical Supplement, 1994.* Washington, D.C.: Government Printing Office.

—————. 1995. *Annual Statistical Supplement to the Social Security Bulletin, 1995.* Washington, D.C.: Government Printing Office.

Wiener, J. 1996. *Can Medicaid Long-Term Care Expenditures for the Elderly by Reduced?* New York: Commonwealth Fund.

Winterbottom, C., D. Liska, and K. Obermaier. 1995. *State-Level Databook on Health Care Access and Financing.* 2d ed. Washington, D.C.: Urban Institute.

13

The Aging Network
A Balancing Act between Universal Coverage and Defined Eligibility

DIANE E. JUSTICE

The Older Americans Act (OAA) defines the primary mission of state and area agencies on aging as developing a comprehensive and coordinated service delivery system for older people. The act embodies values—for example, maximizing the independence of older people, supporting their preferences for receiving long-term care services at home, and empowering consumers with meaningful roles in program governance—that have served as guiding principles in advancing that mission for the aging network since the mid-1970s. And the service funds of the OAA have provided a basic foundation for financing the comprehensive delivery system envisioned in 1965 when the program was enacted.

Beyond these important contributions, however, the act is constrained in its ability to address the most intensive service needs of older people. This constraint is the result of two factors: (1) the obvious mismatch between the program's relatively meager federal resources and its ambitious program goals, and (2) the myth, tenaciously sustained by many federal policy makers and national aging organizations, that the act can actually provide universal access to all older people, regardless of their income or functional need for services. In combination, these factors have yielded a distribution of resources to services that are provided in high volume at relatively low cost per recipient—useful, but thereby limiting the ability of the program to intensively serve those older people who have more complex needs.

Ironically, state agencies on aging have been best able to fulfill the act's vision of a comprehensive delivery system through the use of other resources, ones that reject the OAA philosophy of universal access based solely on age, and instead use explicit eligibility criteria based on both functional and financial needs. Each state now has a Medicaid home and community care waiver program that provides a broad array of services to low-income older people whose disability levels would qualify them for admission to a nursing home. In addition, most states have programs funded by general revenues for people with comparable functional impairments who are required to pay varying portions of their service costs based on their incomes. These types of eligibility policies ensure that public resources are devoted to those most in need, and as a result, governors and state legislatures have been willing to commit substantial resources to home and community services. State and area agencies needed to convince policy makers that the network could judiciously allocate program resources to individuals based on explicit eligibility criteria rather than on the traditional, universal philosophy of the OAA. The delegation of responsibility to state agencies on aging for most programs funded by general revenues and for more than half of the Medicaid waiver programs indicates a recognition that they can be successful in this kind of endeavor.

So, one may ask, why are the paths taken by federal and state policy so different? A comparison of the political context within which the OAA operates at the federal and state levels yields some answers.

The Federal Policy Context

The promise of a universal program capable of serving all older people regardless of their functional status or income holds obvious political appeal. Advocates have increasingly referred to the OAA as an entitlement program, although neither its structure nor its funding level approximates that lofty policy status. As a further indication of the confused perception of the act's status, proposals have been put forth during the past two reauthorizations that would have given older people the right to sue if they were unable to obtain OAA services.

The act provides a listing of priority target populations, which includes low-income minorities and a wide range of other groups— people who are frail, people who live in rural areas, and non-English speakers, among others. Further defining potential program recipients through the establishment of actual individually based eligibility criteria rather than simply listing target populations is a notion that has rarely crept into the implementation of the OAA. Only two references to noneconomic eligibility criteria are made within the act: (1) Title III-C2 home-delivered meals, and (2) Title III-D, a small in-home services program that finances significantly fewer in-home services than does Title III-B, which lacks any reference to functional eligibility criteria. Since neither of these two eligibility references is underscored in congressional committee reports, floor statements, or other documents emphasizing legislative intent, they should not be viewed as a sign that policy makers have embraced the philosophy of defining access to a limited OAA service supply.

States have tried to focus OAA resources on services that help older people who have significant limitations in their ability to conduct activities of daily living. They have done so by using the authority contained in the act that allows states to transfer a certain percentage of funds among service categories. In particular, they have increased spending for home-delivered meals above the amounts appropriated by Congress and decreased spending on congregate meals. However, the political constraints of focusing too extensively on a frail population were underscored by the 1991 reauthorization of the act, which responded to the concerns of congregate meal providers by reducing the amounts available for transfer to home-delivered meals or to any other part of the program.

The extent to which the act should use economic criteria to define consumer need has been the subject of intense and continual debate throughout the evolution of the act (Hudson 1995). Two basic tenets are held by policy makers and advocates, alike: (1) that, in its most colloquial form, the OAA is not a "welfare program" and thus should not use income to determine who should—and should not—receive services, and (2) that services should be targeted to those most in need, with particular attention to low-income minorities. Over time, these principles have come to be viewed as intellectually consistent by many involved with OAA policy—with the notable exception of state and local officials who must implement them.

Given the inability of most policy makers and advocates to come to grips with the limits on the act's resources, it is not surprising that the issue of targeting resources to those in greatest need is framed in a somewhat abstract manner. The formula for the distribution of OAA funds within a state has become the debate's focal point. Legislative language, court cases, and federal regulations have all focused on the question of which demographic factors should be used to allocate service funds among broad geographic areas—all of which avoids the real question of who gets served and, by default, who does not.

During reauthorization debates in both 1987 and 1991, state administrators of the OAA proposed a more specific and direct targeting strategy, which would have given states the option of using consumer cost sharing, through sliding-scale fees based on income, to allocate resources to an individual's service cost. Certain access and advocacy services would have been exempted from sliding-scale fees. People with low incomes would not have been required to share costs; the service costs of others would have been subsidized based on their self-declared income level.

Cost-sharing policies have been used extensively within state-funded home and community care programs as a way of targeting resources based on income without excluding program participants through a means test. In state capitals, these policies received widespread support from consumers, advocates, and state legislators. However, inside the Washington beltway, reactions were quite different. Some advocates thought low-income people would be deterred from participation in OAA programs because they would be unable to understand that cost sharing would not apply to them. Others objected to any consideration of a recipient's income, on the grounds that the OAA would become a "welfare program."

The adoption of cost sharing was proposed during a congressional committee markup of the 1987 amendments to the OAA. Fifteen minutes later, a second set of amendments was introduced that also addressed targeting from the more traditional OAA perspective of referring to priority groups rather than from the perspective of individually based criteria. The committee's reaction to each of these two approaches perfectly characterizes the debate.

The cost-sharing amendment specified that self-declaration of income would be used to calculate cost-sharing rates for program recipients and prohibited the application of cost-sharing policies to people with incomes below 125 percent of the poverty level. After discussing the general principle of using sliding-scale fees based on income, several members suggested that they might consider setting the income floor for the initiation of cost sharing at 300 or 400 percent of the poverty level but certainly not at the level used by most state programs. As either a measure of relative financial need or a criterion for resource allocation, the standard of 300 percent of the poverty level falls far short of reality, since only 20 percent of older people have incomes above that amount. In any event, the majority of committee members did not give serious consideration to the concept, regardless of any particular income level, and therefore the proposal was dead for the 1987 reauthorization cycle.

In contrast, the second set of amendments that was introduced generated overwhelming support and was thought by most members to be a promising solution to this targeting dilemma. All components of the network—states, area agencies, and providers—would be required to set objectives for serving low-income minority older people, to describe in their plans the methods they would use to achieve those objectives, and to report annually on the extent to which the previous year's targets were achieved. Press statements describing the committee's actions that day emphasized the advancements made in increasing targeting under the OAA through the adoption of these amendments. The committee's rejection of the amendment that would have more definitively targeted OAA resources was not mentioned.

By the time reauthorization of the act was considered again in 1991, cost-sharing policies were viewed in a somewhat more favorable light. The U.S. General Accounting Office (1989) had conducted a study mandated by the 1987 amendments and had found positive results from the use of cost sharing by states in other aging programs. While these findings and those of a similar study conducted by the Inspector General's Office of the U.S. Department of Health and Human Services persuaded some to reconsider their previous reluctance to support cost sharing, the preconceptions of many opponents were unchanged. Testifying at a congressional hearing, a witness representing a national aging organization reported learning through an informal survey she conducted of elderly residents of public housing that most of them would not seek OAA services if they were required to declare their incomes. No one questioned how people who would forgo public benefits rather than disclose their incomes had gained access to public housing, illustrating the extent to which this argument of participant deterrence had taken hold. Once again in 1991, cost-sharing policies were not adopted.

The State Policy Context

In the programs administered by the aging network beyond the OAA, the use of needs-based criteria, as opposed to the principle of universal coverage, is rarely debated. Functional need, defined by limitations in conducting activities of daily living, is used extensively in state home and community services programs funded with general revenues and in Medicaid home and community services waivers. This eligibility principle emerged in the late 1970s and early 1980s as states attempted to reduce growth in their Medicaid nursing home budgets by providing care to people living in their own homes who would otherwise require nursing home care. To implement this policy, aging networks established assessment procedures to measure need and determine eligibility, case management systems to develop individual care plans that authorize the amount and type of services to be received by each consumer, and methods for monitoring care plans to ensure that they are being implemented by providers in the manner authorized (Justice 1993).

In the state adult protective services/elder abuse programs, functional need is defined differently. In over half of the states, state agencies on aging administer the adult protective service system, which generally defines its target population as vulnerable adults who are unable to protect themselves from abuse, neglect, or exploitation by others because of a mental or physical impairment. The aging network has responded to this population by establishing administrative structures beyond home and community services programs—to the courts, law enforcement agencies, mental health systems, and guardianship procedures.

Financial need, in aging network programs other than the OAA, is determined through one of two methods, depending on source of funding. In home and community services waiver programs, financial need is obviously a creature of federal Medicaid eligibility policy. Within those limits, states have broad latitude to decide which eligibility options apply to home and community care, such as whether to apply the more generous institutional standard to community care, how much money recipients can retain after becoming eligible for the program, whether spousal impoverishment standards apply, and if people can qualify on the basis of having high medical expenses even if their income exceeds the eligibility threshold.

When state agencies on aging became involved in the administration of home and community services waiver programs, they immersed themselves in the arcane details of this complex web of Medicaid financial eligibility options, both to promote the adoption of state policies that would be most beneficial to older people and to implement the eligibility rules that were ultimately enacted. In comparison, it is fairly straightforward to manage state general revenue programs that use cost sharing based on income. Developed as a way to eliminate income cliffs that lead to all-or-nothing eligibility for Medicaid, cost sharing allows states to serve people of all incomes yet still relate program expenditures to income.

The experiences of state agencies on aging in managing these programs based on functional and financial need led in almost half the states to their management of programs for younger adults with disabilities, further diminishing the principle of universal eligibility based solely on age. In assuming this responsibility, state agencies acquired new names, such as Office of Aging and Adult Services, that reflect their broader mission. But more important, they are now expected in state policy discussions to be the spokesperson for both elderly persons and adults with physical disabilities. Such changes are a somewhat natural evolution of state agencies on aging's role, given the comparable needs for home and community services by these two populations and the absence in many state governments of a focal point for policy coordination on behalf of adults with physical disabilities.

Policy Implications

The aging network has built the comprehensive, coordinated delivery systems envisioned by the Older Americans Act but with non-OAA resources, using functional eligibility criteria, which link income criteria to service support, and increasingly serving younger adults with physical disabilities. Why then has federal OAA policy remained so static? There are three possible reasons, with the first two reflecting differences between federal and state policy perspectives and the third applying to aging programs initiated by both levels of government.

The first factor distinguishing federal and state perspectives on needs-based programs is rooted in the classical principles of federalism, which suggest that policy makers who are in closer proximity to the decisions affecting people's lives are better able to effectively allocate program resources. Decisions made about program populations at the federal level are somewhat abstract, with the individuals they affect removed from direct observation. At the state level, outcomes are more visible. Here, refusing to acknowledge the limits of available funding is less feasible, because the inability of one program to adequately serve its intended recipients places more demand on other related programs. Given this interrelationship between human services programs, setting realistic guidelines for each becomes even more important. Some argue that the real reason that states are more willing to set program eligibility criteria based on functional or financial need is that they are stingy—refusing to fund programs as generously as the federal government. Yet in many states, the level of general revenue funding devoted to aging programs exceeds the state's federal OAA allocations U.S. Administration on Aging 1994).

The second reason for differing perspectives between federal and state officials toward needs-based aging programs lies in the nature of the programs that have historically been under their purview. The major federally administered programs for older people—Social Security and Medicare—are based on a social insurance model, with eligibility based on both age and work history. While both programs have certain features that relate incomes to benefits, they are predominately characterized as universal programs that use age as the sole basis of need. In contrast, the federal programs administered by states are usually means tested; Medicaid, food stamps, and low-income energy assistance are primary examples.

These two distinct program traditions explain a large part of the differing reactions of federal and state policy makers to cost-sharing policies that require people to pay for part of their service costs based on their incomes. Federal officials and national advocacy organizations view cost sharing as a negative departure from universal access based solely on age—even though in the case of the OAA universal access was an unrealized philosophy. State officials and state advocacy groups, on the other hand, view cost sharing as a preferable departure from their means-tested programs, since it provides a vehicle for directly relating benefits to income but avoids denial of service on the basis of income.

A third factor, program size, influences both federal and state policy makers in an identical manner as they consider needs-based policies. In general, it appears more likely that large programs will use needs-based criteria than will smaller ones. This theory seems counterintuitive at first consideration, since lower levels of funding would imply a need for tighter allocation of program resources. However, if a program's budget is significantly less than the amount needed to fulfill its mission, policy makers are likely to conclude that the best political course of action is to avoid defining the size and characteristics of the population to be served. Any further specification of need criteria in this circumstance would either narrow the size of the eligible population to a point that is politically unacceptable or highlight the degree to which program resources are inadequate. Conversely, a more adequate level of funding increases the probability of designing individual need criteria commensurate with available resources. Two examples, one each from federal and state policy, illustrate this point.

The president's health care reform plan, introduced in the fall of 1993, proposed the establishment of a new home and community care program for people of all ages with disabilities. Many of the program's features were drawn from state programs, including the use of functional eligibility based on inability to conduct activities of daily living and requirements for consumers to pay a portion of their care through cost-sharing scales based on income. As was not the case in the OAA debate, neither Congress nor advocacy organizations objected to the inclusion of these program features when the president's plan was discussed. There was some initial concern over the level of need proposed (for example, limitations in at least two or three activities of daily living, percentage of care costs that each income category should be required to pay) but not about the general principle of using these methods to quantify need. When fully implemented, federal funding for this program was expected to reach $36 billion annually. In contrast, OAA funding is a little over $1 billion a year. Neither program provided an individual entitlement that guarantees services to all who meet defined criteria for eligibility. Yet the eligibility criteria included in the president's proposal were consciously structured to match the number of potential program participants with the level of projected program funding.

Likewise, when home and community care programs funded by state general revenue expanded, needs-based eligibility criteria became more, rather than less, rigorous. In the 1970s, these programs mirrored the OAA, combining limited funds with universal eligibility. In the 1980s, as funding increased, states adopted specific eligibility criteria based on ability to perform activities of daily living, which was also the basis for the rapidly expanding Medicaid waiver programs.

The absence of opposition to both the administration's proposed eligibility criteria and comparable factors used in state revenue programs seems to suggest that, once program funding reaches a certain threshold, policy makers and advocates alike begin to realize that resources must be directed to people in need through specific standards. In contrast, policy makers may conclude that establishing functional and income-related criteria for the OAA would only highlight the extent to which its resources fall short of its promise.

Conclusion

The aging network has struggled to accommodate two divergent approaches to targeting the resources of the multiple programs they administer. The more traditional method is based on the universal coverage philosophy of the OAA, which avoids any consideration of individually based need criteria. The other method uses functional eligibility criteria and cost sharing based on income to target scarce resources to those most in need. This latter approach is likely to dominate both federal and state aging services programs as policy makers are forced to respond to the prospects of significantly reduced resources in the years ahead.

References

Hudson, R. 1995. The Older Americans Act and the Defederalization of Community-Based Care. In P. Kim, ed., *Services to Aging and the Aged*. New York: Garland.

Justice, D. 1993. *Case Management Standards in State Community-Based Long-Term Care Programs for Older Persons with Disabilities*. Washington, D.C.: National Association of State Units on Aging.

U.S. Administration on Aging. 1994. *Infrastructure of Home and Community Based Services for the Elderly: A Source Book*. Washington, D.C.

U.S. General Accounting Office. 1989. *In-Home Services for the Elderly: Cost Sharing Expands Range of Services Provided and Population Served*. Washington, D.C.: Government Printing Office.

14

Employer Policy and the Future of Employee Benefits for an Older Population

ANNA M. RAPPAPORT

Traditional employee benefit plans offered by larger employers have been designed with several goals in mind:

• To protect employees and their dependents in the event of medical expenses and against loss of income from death, disability, and retirement.

• To strengthen the ties between company and employee.

• To offer a competitive employment environment.

• To reward career employment.

Plans were designed to allocate benefit dollars more heavily to employees with families and to those who were older, but for many years this fact was largely hidden from employees and not explicitly recognized or discussed by most plan sponsors.

Then in the 1970s, with the growth of health care costs and the emergence of global competition, and in the 1980s, with the growth of flexible benefit plans, employers and employees began to focus more on what was spent and how it was allocated to employee groups. Flexible benefit plans offer a way to let employees take what was being spent for benefits and make various choices. It became obvious that there were subsidies inherent in traditional plans, and many employers sought to reduce them as they changed their benefit structures. At the same time, plan designers had to take into account the fact that the workforce is not homogeneous and that employees vary by family type.

Age and Benefit Design

Age has generally been recognized explicitly in the design of employee benefits. Under traditional benefit designs, costs increase with age, but these costs are generally hidden from employees and often from the plan sponsor as well, since costs are reviewed based on averages for the whole group, rather than as amounts per employee.

There have been, however, a number of public policy initiatives focusing on age and employee benefit management. Age discrimination has been a workplace issue for many years, but benefits generally have not been the focus of this discussion. After 1978, when the Age Discrimination in Employment Act was amended, guidelines have dictated the benefit designs required to avoid age discrimination. Before that point, benefit accruals in defined-benefit retirement plans could be discontinued after normal retirement age. That legislation required employers to continue the accrual of retirement benefits beyond normal retirement age.

The focus of regulations after the 1978 amendments was cost equalization. Employers were allowed to reduce benefits with increases in age as long as costs by age did not discriminate—that is, spending could not decrease with increasing age. The purpose of this rule was to maintain cost-benefit balance so that benefits did not become a disincentive to the hiring of older workers. Traditional retirement benefits encourage employees to stay until retirement. Many employers offer retiree health benefits available only to those who retire from the company. The benefits of the defined-benefit plan also are heavily earned in the years just before retirement, particularly when pay is continuing to increase, and benefits are based on final average earnings.

As employers downsize, they often determine that it would be beneficial to make older employees eligible for early retirement and offer programs that grant additional retirement benefits to those who retire during a temporary "window" of time. As a result of these programs, many workers retire early. There has, however, been litigation regarding age discrimination, and early retirement windows have been one of the concerns. Today, when structuring these windows, employers must address the possibility of age discrimination.

Public Policy and Employer-Sponsored Retirement Benefits

Many requirements are imposed on retirement benefits in the United States, yet public policy is ambivalent toward employer-sponsored retirement benefits. Tax preferences are available through tax-qualified plans to provide retirement benefits to employees as follows: The amounts contributed to tax-qualified plans are not taxed as current income to employees but are subject to income tax when paid out as benefits. In the same way, investment income held in tax-qualified plans is tax deferred, with the money subject to income tax when paid out as benefits. Since the mid-1980s, a growing number of requirements have applied to such plans, with stricter rules and limitation of benefits, particularly for people in higher income brackets. A key principle of recent law has been that benefits may not favor the highly paid.

In fact, because of increasing regulatory requirements, smaller employers have discontinued many of their retirement plans. In addition to a constant stream of new statutory requirements, the enforcement environment has become far more stringent, so practices that were commonplace in the mid-1980s are clearly unacceptable and risky today. Plan sponsors view the public policy environment as adverse to benefits and discouraging to their efforts. Because the need for retirement benefits will increase as the population ages, these are troubling developments.

An example of these difficulties is seen in the case of retirement age provisions in public policy, which generally accept a retirement age range of sixty to sixty-five. While partial Social Security benefits are available as early as sixty-two, the age for the receipt of full benefits is gradually being increased to sixty-seven for people born in 1960. Yet, ERISA (Employee Retirement Income Security Act), a major pension law, does not permit a normal retirement age—that is, retirement with full benefits—later than age sixty-five. One of the key questions of the next few years, then, is whether pension law will be modified to allow a later full-benefit retirement age, to bring pension law and Social Security into synchronization. Without such modifications, workers may be pushed by pension law to retire at age sixty-five but unable to collect full Social Security until age sixty-seven.

The Business Environment and the New Social Contract

Global competition, technology, changing values, and demographics are now encouraging employers to redefine their relationship to their employees. The traditional relationship is built around the paradigm that reasonable performers are secure in their jobs and that the individual can decide whether or not to accept the company's offer of a lifetime job and security. The new paradigm is based on a job that lasts as long as the business supports it, and security has become the responsibility of the individual. Companies are bought and sold, and long-term job security no longer exists. Traditional retirement plans were designed to provide good benefits to career employees—with the notion that employees choose whether to stay or leave early. These plans provide much lower benefits to those who leave early, particularly before early retirement age. Today what is needed is a retirement benefit structure that provides a fair benefit regardless of tenure at termination from each job.

There has been a great deal of focus lately on a "new social contract" or a "changing employment relationship." Under the traditional approach, there is an assumption of job security, that lifetime employment is available to the employee except in the event of very poor performance or some discontinuity in the business (usually seen as an exception, rather than as the norm). A tremendous number of companies since the mid-1980s have gone through changes in ownership, reengineering, and restructuring. The workforces of companies that were once viewed as the bastions of employment stability— traditional banks, telecommunications companies, large steel and auto companies, utilities, and the like—have experienced substantial dislocation. This has led to a focus on a new social contract between employer and employee. Table 14.1 contrasts some of the characteristics of the new and old social contracts.

We can think about the contract as implying different things with respect to how employment terminates and to the period when employment continues.

The Evolving Contract and the Rationale for Termination of Employment

Under the old way of thinking, termination is at the employer's request, for cause or (less common) for poor performance. In addition, it is relatively rare to look carefully at the fit of the individual and the

Table 14.1.
The Traditional and the New Social Contract between Employer
and Employee

Traditional Social Contract	New Social Contract
A growing workforce	Downsizing, rightsizing
Stability	Change and uncertainty
Permanent employees	A mix of permanent and contingent employees
Paternalism and entitlement	Employee responsibility
Retirement as a one-time event	Gradual retirement
Employee retention	Targeted turnover
Job security	Education/skill building to remain employable (at the same place or elsewhere)
Learning at workforce entry	Lifelong learning

job. The individual is free, and often chooses, to leave for a better opportunity, but the option of long-term employment is there. Depending on the organization and the industry, many employees choose long-term employment.

Under the new paradigm, companies are reorganized frequently, and jobs tend to be eliminated if they do not fit the needs of the new organization. Reasons for job termination now include reorganization and downsizing, as well as cause and performance. Organizations are also much more likely to take action on poor performance. The decision regarding whether an employee remains with an organization or leaves is no longer the employee's choice; it is much more often the company's choice.

Under the old paradigm, retirement benefit plans provide high benefits for those who stay until normal retirement age and low benefits for those who leave very early or in their middle years. That structure was once not a problem, since those who left early did so based on their own choice. Today, this pattern poses a problem.

The Evolving Contract and Periods of Continued Employment

Under the old way of thinking, planning and expecting change are not part of the social fabric; under the new way of thinking, change is to be expected and is part of the environment. Under the old way of thinking, although there is ongoing training, its importance to the individual or to the company is not recognized; under the new way of thinking, maintaining human capital is a major issue for both employee and employer. Under the old way of thinking, there is structure and hierarchy; under the new way of thinking, there is a much less hierarchy. The evolution of the contract means that pay systems need to be more flexible, to include a higher component of incentive compensation.

The transition to a different culture is difficult for both employees and employers. For employees over age forty-five with long service, this transition is particularly difficult, since many of these employees built their lives based on expectations that grew out of the old culture and a different social contract. One human resources officer, in looking at the accrual pattern under a traditional defined-benefit plan, expressed the needs of the new environment with two statements: "We need to offer a plan such that if an employee leaves at any point in time we are square and treat the employee fairly," and "We need to protect our employees in the event we are acquired. In our industry, 25 percent to 33 percent of the employees will usually lose their jobs after an acquisition." That human resources officer was very uncomfortable with the traditional defined-benefit plan, with its steep accrual pattern.

Traditional Retirement Plans: Do They Work Today?

Traditional retirement plans include defined-benefit plans and defined-contribution plans. The traditional defined-benefit plan uses a final average earnings formula, so that benefits are a percentage multiplied by years of service and average earnings in the final five years of employment. In contrast, defined-contribution plans offer an individual account based on amounts credited to the employee's account plus interest.

The relevance of traditional plans is not a new subject. The death of defined-benefit plans has been declared periodically since the 1940s because (1) they are old-fashioned and complex, (2) younger employees do not appreciate them, and (3) they are risky. Nevertheless, larger employers (those with over a thousand employees) have continued these plans. There has been little change in their frequency of use, even though the number of employees covered has declined as employment patterns have shifted. The principal reasons for this are that they are efficient and that their risks carry rewards. For those employees who stay until retirement, these plans deliver the most dollars for employer dollars invested (the goal of many employers). And employers who have managed their assets well have been well rewarded for taking that risk.

Plan Choices of the 1990s

For those employers who believe the old options do not work well today, new options supplement traditional defined-benefit and defined-contribution plans. Hybrid plans offer features of both. The cash balance plan is a defined-benefit plan in which the benefit is defined as an account within the plan. The plan specifies the rates of contribution and investment return (independent of plan asset performance) to be credited to the participant's account. This plan looks like a defined-contribution plan for the purposes of benefit accrual. The target benefit plan is a defined-contribution plan in which the benefit is calculated to reproduce the benefits in a defined-benefit formula. The benefit accrual pattern in this type of plan is more like a defined-benefit plan. Table 14.2 shows the characteristics of hybrid cash balance plans, traditional defined-benefit plans, and traditional defined-contribution plans.

Table 14.2.
Traditional and Hybrid Benefit Plans

Characteristic	Traditional Defined Benefit	Hybrid Cash Balances	Traditional Defined Contribution
Allocation of dollars	Heavily to years of later service	Heavier to early years of service (can modify with formula)	Heavily to early years of service
Bearer of investment risk	Employer	Employer	Employee
Ability to grandfather in prior defined-benefit formula inside	Yes	Yes	No
Ability to offer early retirement windows inside plan	Yes	Yes	No
Investment choices available to employees	No	No	Yes
Ability to vary accruals by age and length of service	Formula does automatically (but not obvious)	Yes, subject to passing non-discrimiation tests	Yes, subject to passing non-discrimiation tests
Can base benefits on profits	No	No	Yes
Bearer of inflation risk	Usually employer	Employee	Employee

Traditional defined-benefit (final average earnings) plans, which provide for heavy benefit accruals late in the employee's career, are in line with the old social contract, whereas defined-contribution plans based on cash balance designs provide for much heavier benefit accruals earlier and, therefore, fit better with the new employer-employee relationship. Traditional defined-benefit plans usually offer payout as a monthly income, fitting the entitlement orientation of the old social contract, whereas cash balance and defined-contribution plans usually offer payout as lump sums, more in line with the new contract. All plan types can offer other forms of payout as options.

Many Americans do not have the skills or the interest in saving and financial planning that are required to develop and execute a regular program of savings. For them, the new environment is a major challenge. They need to save early, to plan, and to be able to evaluate options. Some employers offer support for financial planning, but these are relatively few. With personal computers, however, new options are available to employees at modest cost, and employers can be expected to encourage employees in their financial and retirement planning through educational programs.

Change is the main characteristic of the 1990s, with the evolving social contract between employer and employee an important example. Change is reflected in organizational structure, culture, compensation, and benefits. The playout of these issues will have a substantial impact on policy toward older workers. As a result of such ongoing change, many employers are reexamining their retirement strategies. The questions they are asking include, Why do we offer this program? Do we get value from it? Is it a good way to spend our money? The environment and the emphasis have shifted. I predict the following changes in the retirement package:

• An increase in employee responsibility for retirement. Financial planning at the personal level will be much more widespread. Retirement security will depend heavily on what the individual has done about planning.

• A reduction in employer coverage for medical care for Medicare-eligible retirees and an increase in employee contributions toward health care at any age.

• An increased focus on Medicare risk contracts as a way to cover retiree health care.

• A decline in employer-provided benefits for all and a shift to matched savings programs, which focus on employee responsibility.

• A redesign of many pension plans to a cash balance or other approach that modifies the benefit accrual pattern while retaining the employer investment risk and the favorable returns that can accrue from risk assumption.

• An increased choice in investment options in employee savings programs and more savings education.

• A continued focus on early retirement windows and reductions in subsidies in nonwindow situations.

• More options for gradual retirement.

• A gradual increase in full retirement age.

• Continued corporate restructuring and the accompanying elimination of jobs.

• An increase in second and third careers.

As the workforce and social contract change, total retirement program design, as well as pension plan design, will need to be revisited. Employees will have more responsibility, and a new type of partnership between employer and employee will emerge.

References

American Compensation Association. ACA *Journal, Perspectives in Compensation and Benefits, ACA News,* books on benefits topics.

Employee Benefit Research Institute. Databook, issue briefs, and special books on employee benefit topics.

International Foundation of Employee Benefit Plans. *Employee Benefits Journal, Benefits Quarterly.*

Pension Research Council. Books and occasional papers on benefits topics.

Society of Actuaries. *North American Actuarial Journal, the Actuary, Pension Section News, Health Section News.*

U.S. Chamber of Commerce. *Employee Benefits Sourcebook.* Annual survey of cost and use of employee benefits.

U.S. Department of Labor. Periodic surveys of use of benefits.

PART IV

TWO CASE STUDIES

15

Funding Elder Home Care from the Bottom Up
Policy Choices for a Local Community

ROBERT LOGAN and
ROBERT APPLEBAUM

On November 3, 1992, the citizens of Hamilton County, Ohio, did something unusual: voters approved a $13 million-a-year property tax levy designed to fund in-home services for older residents. As a result, the Elderly Services Program (ESP), administered by the Cincinnati Council on Aging (one of twelve regional area agencies on aging in Ohio), currently serves more than 4,700 county residents needing in-home care. With a triage model, the program uses multiple levels of care management to authorize and monitor the in-home services provided. This chapter describes the policy issues and choices examined as ESP went from a proposal for expanding in-home care to an actual operating services program funded by the electorate.

Background

The impetus for the in-home program in Hamilton County mirrors the national concern about the lack of services available to older people requesting care outside of a nursing home setting. County agencies serving older people and their families repeatedly described the limited availability and affordability of in-home care. As in most communities, funds from the Older Americans Act, the Social Services Block Grant, and the United Way were being reduced or remaining level while the frail aged population was growing.

The state of Ohio had developed a large in-home care program funded through the Medicaid waiver (termed PASSPORT). However, fiscal constraints, severe restrictions on income and assets, and strict entry criteria made the program available to only a small proportion (5%) of Hamilton County's older population. Growing waiting lists for in-home care inspired the commitment to expand in-home services through the proposed levy.

The idea for tax-levy funding has its roots in two phenomena. Hamilton County has a history of supporting social service programs through similar types of efforts. By 1992, voters had approved additional taxes to support a county rehabilitation hospital, medical care for low-income persons, services for developmentally disabled individuals, mental health services, children's services, and on the lighter side, the Cincinnati Zoo. The total amount raised for the above programs was more than $132 million. The second phenomenon that supported the proposed effort was the success of a similar levy in another part of the state (Columbus, Franklin County). Consideration of the property tax in Hamilton County raised two policy questions: Is local government the appropriate entity to fund long-term care services? And is the property tax an appropriate mechanism for raising revenues for such a program?

An editorial in the major daily newspaper (the *Cincinnati Enquirer*, Oct. 14, 1992) summed up the policy debate faced by communities.

> Each designated tax makes it that much harder to pass levies for schools and other purposes. Yes, the elderly need help; but so do children, who are about three times more likely to live poverty. The nationwide poverty rate for the elderly is less than 12 percent; for children in Cincinnati, it's 37 percent. Child abuse cases multiplied by 10 between 1975 and 1991. . . . Nonetheless, we support the levy for the elderly for several reasons:
>
> • Such targeted taxes are a good way to get more bang for the buck by keeping spending under local control.
>
> • It's a way for voters to make sure money is spent on the specific purposes they support.
>
> • It can be justified as a money saver if it reduces costs for elderly care and eases the burden on families.
>
> • And it has a five-year expiration date. The tax ends in 1996, when we can review it before we renew it.
>
>   Let's face it: government leaders who leave it up to the taxpayers to pick and choose from a menu of worthy causes are ducking their respon-

sibility to set priorities for spending. Care for the elderly—and children—gets too little attention. If government can't do the job with all the taxes it collects, voters will have to do it themselves. We support Issue 6.

Thus, while there were differences in philosophy about the use of the property tax to finance the program, from a pragmatic perspective, there were few options, and given the historical precedent, the approach was approved.

Issues of Program Design

The development of any health and social service program includes myriad policy choices. When coupled with a financing scheme that entails voter approval of a tax levy, such decisions become magnified. In addition to questions of financing, three program design issues were identified for policy debate: age criteria, income criteria, and level-of-disability criteria.

Age Criteria

One of the most controversial national policy issues in the long-term care reform debate centers on the question of whether long-term care systems should be designed differently for varying age groups. On the one hand, policy analysts have argued that long-term care involves assistance to individuals with functional limitations and that such services are not age related. On the other hand, the service network approach to long-term care has varied by group. For example, home care for older people has relied heavily on the use of case managers, but younger physically disabled people have typically expressed an interest in managing their own care. Programs for older people have typically used agency-based in-home workers, while many younger physically disabled individuals report a preference for hiring and supervising their own workers. Are these differences real? And do such differences result in legitimate reasons to separate community long-term care programs on the basis of age? Unfortunately, empirical research has not addressed these policy issues.

Although such a debate raises many difficult questions, the decision was actually relatively straightforward for the levy program because the lead organizations involved in the levy campaign are agencies of the aging network. The choice to direct the program to those over age sixty was without major controversy. The over-sixty population was the group with which the lead agencies had experience and expertise, so an age-based plan allowed them to concentrate on their area of strength. This network had worked together as a group during the Pew Foundation Living at Home program. The model for the initiative was a state demonstration developed by the Ohio Department of Aging for the over-sixty population, and as in most communities, the aging network and the physically disabled, mental health, and developmental disabilities networks had not established strong working relationships. Finally, the services program for mental health and the developmentally disabled were actually funded by an existing levy.

Income Criteria

Because long-term care services are financed by a range of funding sources, state and federal policy on income eligibility has been at best inconsistent and at worst plagued by conflict. Home care funded under the 2176 Medicaid waiver has had strict requirements for income and assets. Home care paid for through the Older Americans Act, although targeted toward lower- and moderate-income groups, is generally not income tested. The Social Services Block Grant and state-funded home care programs have been targeted toward groups in between these two groups. The Medicare home health component operates on a social insurance model. It provides coverage for acute illnesses and also in-home services to many chronically disabled older people. The long-term care piece of the now-defunct Health Security Act included benefits for low- and moderate-income individuals, who could pay through the use of a sliding scale.

Professional experience and politics both contributed to the ESP position on income eligibility. Agencies had been continually frustrated by the strict limitations on income and assets under Medicaid. Although many state home care waiver programs allow income eligibility to be increased to between 200 percent and 300 percent of the Supplemental Security Income (SSI) program (between $850 and $1,300 per month), states are unable to modify the asset requirement. Since many older people have some private savings, the $1,500 limitation excludes a large proportion of the older population. Agency personnel believed that many low- and moderate-income people needed in-home assistance but were unable receive such care under the waiver program.

A political rationale also influenced the policy discussion in this area. With the levy requiring approval from the electorate, organizers did not want the public to view this as a program targeted toward a small segment of the older population. The program proposed a model in which intake, referral, and case management were to be performed regardless of income, while payment for services would be based on a sliding scale. Specific dollar amounts were not established until after the passage of the levy. Currently, about one-third of the service recipients have incomes over 150 percent of the poverty level, the point at which individuals are required to share in the costs of service. Because some health and service expenditures are exempt from the income calculations, about 13 percent of clients actually are required to share the cost.

Level of Disability

Home care programs have also had to address questions about the level of disability of care recipients. Medicaid waiver programs, as well as the vast majority of state-funded home care programs, have targeted in-home care toward the most disabled population. For example, the waiver home care programs require that recipients be at the level of residents of a nursing home intermediate-care facility. With very limited dollars it is certainly reasonable to target care toward highly disabled people. This practice, however, results in lack of access to the formal care system for many moderately impaired people. The staffs of agencies in the network believe that a number of older people, particularly those living alone, have moderate limitations requiring them to need assistance. Recognizing that some of this care might prove to be preventive in nature, program organizers believe that some home care funds should be allocated for moderately impaired persons. Additionally, funds are to be allocated for a wider range of services than those provided by the traditional service network. These services include home repair and modification, equipment and supplies, and legal services. About 20 percent of the care recipients in the program receive assistance in this category.

Implementation Experience

ESP has completed its second year of program operations. With more than five thousand care recipients, the program has considerably more enrollees than the nine hundred people participating in the state Medicaid waiver program. A comparison of ESP and the home care waiver program provides some insights into the similarities and differences in

Table 15.1.
The ESP Levy Program and the PASSPORT Medicaid Waiver Program

Characteristic	ESP	PASSPORT
Age (%)		
60–65	5.2	13.6
66–74	29.7	26.2
75–84	42.7	38.6
85–90	15.9	15.9
91+	7.3	5.7
Race (%)		
Caucasian	65.9	65.5
Noncaucasian	34.1	34.5
Gender (%)		
Female	78.2	77.5
Male	21.8	22.5
Marital status (%)		
Married	24.4	17.0
Nonmarried	75.6	83.0
Income 150 percent of poverty		
or below (%)	59.0	98.0
ADL impairments (%)		
0	22.5	0.5
1	18.3	5.5
2	16.1	31.0
3	12.9	29.0
4 or more	30.2	34.0
Cost per person ($)	253	660

the structure and nature of the two efforts. As shown in table 15.1 the demographic profiles of the two programs are comparable, with age, race, and gender being quite similar. Reflecting the differences in income eligibility, ESP clients, while generally of low-income status, are less likely to be below poverty than almost all of the Medicaid program participants. Marital status and income are linked and, as expected, ESP has a higher proportion of married clients than those in the Medicaid waiver program.

The disability profile of program participants highlights the differences between the two programs. The Medicaid waiver program is designed to serve those at risk of placement in a nursing home. Thus, the vast majority of waiver clients have substantial functional disability. For example, 94 percent had two or more limitations in activities of daily living (ADL) and 63 percent had three or more limitations. In comparison, 41 percent of ESP clients had one or no ADL limitation, although most have multiple limitations in instrumental activities of daily living (IADL; e.g., doing housework, shopping). One segment of the ESP caseload, however, is highly disabled, with more than 30 percent of clients reporting four or more ADL limitations. These differences are reflected in the costs of care, with ESP averaging $253 per month, compared to $660 for the Medicaid waiver program.

The levy allows the agency to diverge from the Medicaid waiver in two important ways. First, although the program continues to serve low-income older people, it also serves some low- and moderate-income older people who have been traditionally excluded from Medicaid. A big part of the reason for this is that the Medicaid waiver uses the limited asset requirement ($1,500 per individual), which is not used in ESP. Many low-income clients, despite being income eligible, are ineligible because of the Medicaid asset rule. The second difference involves disability criteria. As a nursing home alternative, the Medicaid waiver clients must meet nursing home level-of-care criteria. Although about 40 percent of ESP clients meet this criterion, many are in much earlier stages of disability. Clinical staff argue that a strength of the program lies in its preventive aspect, allowing it to serve clients across the disability spectrum.

The effect of these changes is that the ESP has enrolled a substantial number of older people. By early 1997 the program had enrolled 5,500 people, compared to about 900 Medicaid waiver participants. Many policy questions are raised as a result of such an intervention. For example, how can we balance the desire to make home care available to older people who have a range of disabilities in the context of limited budget growth? The demand for ESP enrollment has been substantial and, even with considerable resources, the program will be unable to meet all requests. With limited resources, how should care be allocated: by level of disability, type of service, or income? The Medicaid waiver programs around the nation have targeted care toward those with the greatest level of disability and the lowest incomes and thus have not had to extend the debate any further. Programs such as ESP have thus entered uncharted waters in struggling with these difficult allocational decisions.

Decisions about criteria for eligibility appear to be reinforced by practical experience. There has been little discussion about serving the under-sixty population, although funding from a private foundation was recently received to explore the issues facing the population of all disabled individuals. The cost-sharing component has generated very little controversy. The vast majority of enrollees pay nothing according to the sliding-scale fee formula, and those who are required to pay have not expressed reluctance to contribute. Finally, network agencies and program staff affirmed the decision about level of disability, and both groups identify the ability to serve a moderately impaired population as important for a community program. The levy goes back to voters in 1997. That vote will be the ultimate test of the strategy and its overall implementation.

16

The State of California Linkages Program
Focus on Functional Status

MONIKA WHITE

In the early 1980s, the development of a California state plan on long-term care was under way. Originally conceptualized as a gap-filling initiative for elderly persons not eligible for existing programs, the effort soon became the focus of heated discussion and active lobbying as advocates for both senior and disabled persons debated the issues. Discussions centered on how to achieve a continuum of care, where the program should be located, and who should be served.

At the time, the state's 2176 Medicaid waiver program, the Multi-Purpose Senior Services Program (MSSP), had already been moved from demonstration to ongoing program status and had grown from eight to twenty-two sites. Through a combination of purchased and referred services coordinated by case managers, the program provided alternatives to nursing home care for people who were frail, age sixty-five or older, eligible for Medicaid, certified for placement in a skilled or intermediate-care facility, and living in specific geographic areas. Other programs such as social and health day care centers for older adults and independent living centers for disabled persons were growing to serve populations at risk. Still, the so-called long-term care system, ranging from home and community support services like transportation and personal care to nursing home care, was characterized by fragmentation and duplication.

The case management approach used in MSSP appeared to work well in enhancing access to existing public and private resources and in advocating for client needs. The ability to purchase services with Medicaid funds, in combination with referrals to other local publicly funded and informal services, greatly expanded the options MSSP case managers had to keep their clients at home. But eligibility for MSSP was rigidly defined by the waiver—as to not only who could be served but also the total number that could be served annually throughout the state. As a result, the program did not begin to reach all those in need, since the multiple criteria of age, income, location, and frailty all had to be met at once.

There was a growing recognition that many individuals not eligible for MSSP needed the same access to services and were at risk of institutionalization in their absence. Wouldn't it be nice if there was a program with enough flexibility to begin where MSSP left off? Wouldn't it be nice if a forty-three-year-old who met all MSSP criteria but age or a ninety-two-year-old who did not receive Medicaid could benefit from the expertise of a case manager and access to community resources? Wouldn't it be nice if people could get help even for a short period of time or until a problem is solved? Many community leaders serving elderly people in the community thought so. So did those working with disabled people. Senior groups and advocates for disabled persons mobilized to broaden access to long-term care services statewide.

The State of California Health Department applied for additional Medicaid waivers but was unsuccessful in obtaining them. Interest and lobbying activities nonetheless remained strong, and the pressure was on to develop a statewide long-term care plan without funding or waivers from the outside. The California Department on Aging (CDA), other state departments, area agencies on aging, independent living centers, other community service agencies, and disabled consumers mounted a concerted advocacy effort. Letters were written, vignettes were collected and presented, and strong lobbying activities were undertaken in Sacramento. Finally, it was determined that California would have a program serving multiple populations, providing case management for both short-term and long-term care, and focusing on low-income people without being exclusively targeted toward them. These ingredients were critical to the success of a program designed expressly to meet the needs of individuals not being served by other state programs or services.

Program Design

The program established by the state legislature in 1984 to be administered by the California Department on Aging was designated Linkages. The legislation states that the Linkages program is part of the state's efforts to further "the incremental development of a long-term care delivery system that provides the social and health support necessary to enable frail elderly and functionally impaired adults to remain in their own homes." The program is funded through state general funds, and its purpose is to prevent or delay institutionalization by linking individuals to providers of home and community services through comprehensive information and assistance and case management. The principal linkage, if you will, was to be the functional status of clients to the appropriate array of nonmedical service assistance.

Ten sites were initially selected to administer the programs, and three others were added later. For the first five years, each of the thirteen sites served two hundred clients, with the number then reduced to one hundred clients. Initially, the program set minimal standards, requiring that clientele consist of at least 25 percent non-Medicaid elderly and 25 percent younger disabled people. It had been hoped that funds would be available to purchase services, as was the case with MSSP, but this was not to be the case. However, Linkages was designed so that eligibility criteria were quite flexible. Elderly people regardless of income and younger people with disabilities could get help in identifying problems and needs, locating services, and coordinating resources. Information and referral services were to be available by telephone.

The decision to include both elderly and younger disabled people was based on the recognition that long-term care needs were not limited to elderly persons—that many younger disabled persons were also unable to gain access to needed care. A number of issues arose related to mixing these populations in one program. First, there were strong feelings that the needs of elderly and disabled persons differed significantly and that the resources needed were totally separate. There was also a belief that case managers needed different knowledge bases and different sets of skills to work with these different populations. Finally, there were concerns that one population would take resources from the other. However, none of these matters proved to be a barrier to the success of the program.

Implementation of the Program

Since 1990, the Linkages program has served between 2,000 and 2,200 unduplicated clients annually on a statewide basis. (Before a reduction in the program in 1989–90, twice as many were served.) In 1991 the majority of Linkages clients were Caucasian women (72%), over sixty years of age (80%), living alone (52%), and receiving Medi-Cal (54%; CDA 1991, 7). Since 1991, reporting requirements have changed; however, according to a CDA staff member, client, service, and cost data remain comparable; a 1996 telephone survey conducted by CDA shows an increase in clients under age sixty, from 20 percent in 1991 to 31 percent in 1996. All clients are at risk of institutionalization by virtue of requiring help with one or more activities of daily living as determined by a functional assessment.

Linkages provides three types of service: information only, information with referral, and case management. Arrangement of services from other resources is a key function of the program. Those most frequently arranged are in-home services, transportation, housing, and meals. Among those most often purchased are emergency response systems (CDA 1991, 8). The primary sources of referrals are home health agencies, hospitals for acute illness care, and family members. Other sources include senior centers, MSSP, and county social service departments (ibid.). Individuals eligible for other California state department programs, such as mental health, rehabilitation, or developmental services, may not be enrolled in Linkages.

Total Linkages expenditures for 1994–95 were nearly $2.8 million, including about $1.9 million state general funds, $700,000 local service cash, and $124,000 in-kind contributions. This translates into approximately $116 per client per month. In comparison, MSSP costs ran about $20.4 million for 5,900 unduplicated clients, or $293 per client per month for the same year. The difference is due to MSSP's direct purchase of services as well as the inclusion of all public service expenditures in client cost calculations.

Because of its intentionally flexibility provisions regarding eligibility and length of service and its focus on meeting needs without using "effectiveness" as the principal outcome criterion, Linkages continues to fill important client and service gaps along the continuum of care. The program has also proven to be cost-effective, operating with no budget increases since 1991, while continuing to serve the same numbers of clients. The challenges to Linkages have been in defining its services, setting quality standards, establishing procedures and reporting formats, and managing information. The low likelihood of increased funding in coming years will impede further progress.

New Directions

Because of state funding problems, new directions have been set for the Linkages program. First, it now appears that its the future will lie in the hands of California's counties. Some counties, including San Diego, San Mateo, and Los Angeles, have provided financial support for its Linkages programs for several years. Los Angeles County, for example, allocates a small percentage of the fines it collects for illegal parking in handicapped parking spaces to the Linkages sites in the county. This practice has enabled the sites to offset some increasing costs. The development of state and local partnerships, as exemplified by Linkages, is evidence of the belief in and support for the program.

Through the success of Linkages, service and advocacy groups in California have demonstrated the ability to carry forward the commitment to serving an estimated 2.5 million adults statewide in need of long-term care through one system. During the spring of 1996, a consortium of groups (the California Association of Area Agencies on Aging, the California Commission on Aging, the California Foundation for Independent Living Centers, the California Senior Legislature, the Public Interest Center on Long-Term Care, and the Triple A Council of California) reprinted a paper originally published in January 1995 entitled "A Call for the Development and Restructuring of California's Long-Term Care System." The paper challenges California to make long-term care a top priority, calls for a reorganization of its fragmented system and its categorical services and for the integration of health and social services funding, and delineates strategies for implementing a new system by the year 2000.

The document argues that "long-term care services for both younger and older adults are similar and frequently provided to both groups by the same agencies. California can ill afford to maintain its current duplicate service systems for these two age groups. We urge the creation of a system for the delivery of long-term care services to adults age 18 and above who require assistance with an activity of daily living to live independently. Inappropriate or premature institutionalization must be avoided."

The Future

Efforts to create a single system of care for adults in need of long-term care have resulted in legislation directing the movement of several adult programs supported with state general funds, including Linkages, to county-level area agencies on aging. As of September 1996, the bill was on the governor's desk. If passed, the law would have taken effect on January 1, 1997, and monies from the general funds as well as management responsibilities for the designated programs would be transferred to the area agencies on aging. Services may be provided directly by the county or through contracts with local agencies. While some uneasiness exists among local service providers about the potential impact of these changes, the current shift toward local control seems to pose no immediate threat to the continued development and maintenance of a long-term care system that serves multiple adult populations.

Linkages has become a strong and positive part of the community long-term care system in California. The movement away from serving only frail elderly persons toward serving multiple functionally impaired populations has gained widespread acceptance. Linkages is generally seen as a successful program in both aging and disability networks. There is every indication that the underlying policy decisions about long-term care made by California's legislature in the early 1980s will continue to shape service delivery for the state's functionally impaired adult populations for some time to come.

Reference

CDA (California Department on Aging, Long-Term Care and Aging Services Division). 1991. *Report to the Legislature.* March.

Index

Library of Congress Cataloging-in-Publication Data

The future of age-based public policy / edited by Robert B. Hudson.
  p. cm.
Includes bibliographical references and index.
ISBN 0-8018-5659-0 (alk. paper). — ISBN 0-8018-5660-4 (pbk. : alk. paper)
  1. Old age assistance—United States. 2. Aged—Government policy—United States. I. Hudson, Robert B., 1944–
HV1461.F88 1997
362.6'3—dc21   97-5476   CIP